COMPETENCY ASSESSMENT

A Practical Guide to the Joint Commission Standards

Third Edition

Brenda G. Summers
MBA/MHA, MSN, RN, CNAA-BC

WendySue Woods
RN, CSHA, MHSA

HCPro

Competency Assessment: A Practical Guide to the Joint Commission Standards, Third Edition, is published by HCPro, Inc.

Copyright © 2008, 2004, 2001 HCPro, Inc.

All rights reserved. Printed in the United States of America.   5 4 3 2 1

First edition published 2001. Second edition 2004. Third edition 2008.

ISBN # 978-1-60146-251-0

No part of this publication may be reproduced, in any form or by any means, without prior written consent of HCPro, Inc., or the Copyright Clearance Center (978/750-8400). Please notify us immediately if you have received an unauthorized copy.

HCPro, Inc., provides information resources for the healthcare industry.

HCPro, Inc., is not affiliated in any way with The Joint Commission, which owns the JCAHO and Joint Commission trademarks.

Brenda G. Summers, MBA/MHA, MSN, RN, CNAA-BC, Author	Paul Singer, Layout Artist
WendySue Woods, RN, CSHA, MHSA, Author	Matthew Kuhrt, Copyeditor
Jay Kumar, Editor	Sada Preisch, Proofreader
Brian Driscoll, Executive Editor	Darren Kelly, Books Production Supervisor
John Novack, Group Publisher	Susan Darbyshire, Art Director
Jackie Diehl Singer, Graphic Artist	Jean St. Pierre, Director of Operations

Advice given is general. Readers should consult professional counsel for specific legal, ethical, or clinical questions.

Arrangements can be made for quantity discounts. For more information, contact:

HCPro, Inc.
P.O. Box 1168
Marblehead, MA 01945
Telephone: 800/650-6787 or 781/639-1872
Fax: 781/639-2982
E-mail: *customerservice@hcpro.com*

Visit HCPro at its World Wide Web sites:
www.hcpro.com and *www.hcmarketplace.com*

Contents

About the authors..v
Preface..vii

Chapter 1: Competency basics 1
    Definitions and examples of low-volume/high-risk, new or changed,
    problem-prone, and mandated duties 8

Chapter 2: Competency assessments and the Joint
Commission standards..17
    Competency assessment tool 35

Chapter 3: Six steps to a successful competency program 37
    Example of portion of department-specific guidelines 50
    Sampling of population-specific components 51
    Review process categories 57
    Hospitalwide medication errors 59
    Fourth floor medication errors 59
    Fourth floor medication errors by type and shift 60
    Sample questions for self-assessment of motivation 63

Chapter 4: What is the competency validation cycle? 67

Chapter 5: What are validation methodologies? 81
    Validation methodologies and the dimensions of competency they measure............86

Chapter 6: Ongoing measure of core competency..97
    Analyzing medication error data 103
    Aggregated medication error data 104

Contents

Chapter 7: The competency validation process **107**
    Competency validation process 110
    Applicant worksheet 111
    Registered nurse job description 114
    Registered radiologic technologist job description 120
    Security officer job description 126
    Ongoing competency assessment, Sample 1 130
    Ongoing competency assessment, Sample 2 131
    Ongoing competency assessment, Sample 3 132
    Annual performance evaluation: Organizational competencies 133

Chapter 8: Managing the competency program **139**
    Ongoing competency statement 144
    Competency Management Council 146

About the authors

WendySue Woods

WendySue Woods, RN, CSHA, MHSA, brings exceptional accreditation compliance and process improvement expertise to her clients. She has more than 20 years of consulting experience and frontline, real-time success in Joint Commission accreditation, regulatory/risk management compliance, medical staff leadership, process improvement strategies, customer service, and administrative facility operations.

Prior to becoming a full-time consultant for The Greeley Company, Woods served in varying hospital administration roles related to quality management and medical staff leadership. She has successfully led organizations to Joint Commission accreditation compliance, achieving accreditation without recommendations for improvement. Woods served as Administrator of Operations and Ancillary Services for a hospital-owned, Joint Commission-accredited physician group. Her customer satisfaction programs have resulted in increased annual scores and greater market share. Her varied experience and ability to understand compliance, implement process improvement strategies across all levels, and provide staff education across the continuum, bring a comprehensive and realistic approach to reengineering and regulatory compliance.

Woods' ease with her clients and audience allows organizations to better understand the value of process improvement, customer service, and regulatory compliance and gain the ability to incorporate it into daily operations. She brings enthusiasm and a practical approach to healthcare accreditation. She has addressed healthcare audiences throughout the Southeast on topics varying from medical staff leadership, organizational improvement, team building, and Joint Commission accreditation. Woods is a registered nurse and also holds a master's degree in health science administration.

Brenda G. Summers

Brenda G. Summers, MBA/MHA, MSN, RN, CNAA-BC, is a senior consultant with The Greeley Company of Marblehead, MA, focusing on the areas of accreditation and regulatory compliance. She brings more than 16 years of experience in healthcare leadership to her work with healthcare centers across the country. Summers applies her years of healthcare leadership and clinical and regulatory expertise to help clients understand and meet accreditation standards and compliance expectations. Her in-depth understanding of organizational dynamics and the nature of change, even in times of turbulence, allows her to bring a realistic approach to organizational problem solving and strategic and operational process design.

She presents at state and national seminars, participates in topical audio conferences, and has authored several trade publications. Summers has particular expertise in the area of effective competence validation and performance review processes redesign, and consults in all areas of accreditation and regulatory compliance, process improvement, sustained change, and effective models for education.

Prior to joining The Greeley Company, Summers held senior leadership positions in hospitals in both North and South Carolina. Immediately prior to joining The Greeley Company, she served as vice president for administration and chief nursing officer for The Mercy Hospitals in Charlotte, North Carolina. She had direct reporting responsibility for all patient care areas, as well as many other clinical and non-clinical departments of the organization. She successfully introduced a number of change initiatives that resulted in improved patient, staff, and physician satisfaction, improved patient outcomes, and financial success of the organization. While in her senior leadership position, she also had responsibility for accreditation and regulatory affairs for the organization, and was able to coordinate sustained compliance activities in these arenas.

Summers holds an MBA/MHA from Pfeiffer University. She received a B.S. and M.S. in nursing from the University of North Carolina, Chapel Hill. She is certified by the ANCC in Nursing Administration, Advanced and is a member of Sigma Theta Tau, the International Honor Society of Nursing.

Preface

Complying with The Joint Commission (TJC) standards and maintaining accreditation can be challenging, time consuming, and frustrating. It's not uncommon to hear staff in healthcare facilities complain that the time they spend dealing with compliance issues and survey preparation takes away from their top priority: caring for patients. In some instances, staff members are just expressing their frustrations, but in others, they have lost sight of one important fact: Joint Commission standards are intended to promote safe, effective patient care.

Once organizations begin to view TJC standards as a vehicle for maintaining and improving quality of care and patient safety, they're likely to spend less time reading the fine print in their accreditation manual and more time talking about what's best for patients. Organizations should not assess competency simply because a regulatory body mandates it be done. Competency assessment should bring value to the patient, the employee, and the organization. It is a critical component of any process design or redesign, whether in response to opportunities identified through the facility's internal monitoring and evaluation activities or directed by an external source.

Competency assessment does not have to be a laborious, repetitive, paper-only process. Organizations should design a process that is both efficient and meaningful, and when appropriate, fun and memorable. To streamline the process and give it meaning, organizations should embrace the synergy between human resources (HR) and the environment of care (EC), infection control (IC), and performance improvement (PI) functions, and use aggregate data from all these sources.

Today, healthcare leaders are challenged to lay a firm foundation for competency assessment and implement an ongoing and interactive verification of knowledge and skills, while promoting a culture of safety. The goal is to provide high-quality patient care through skilled, competent personnel whose competency is validated and maintained via a structured program. This book provides organizations with the essential definitions and tools they need to understand competency assessment requirements and develop and implement effective competency assessment programs in their facilities. It has been updated to address competency as it relates to tracer methodology, the evaluation of orientation, and the process for competence validation. We provide a model for competency validation and discuss the six steps to a successful program. A detailed discussion of the role data can play in the assessment of ongoing competence is also included.

Chapter One

Competency Basics

Competency basics

Establishing and implementing a thorough and effective, competency assessment program is the key to complying with the Joint Commission's (TJC's) competency-related standards. A competency assessment program should focus on identifying, verifying, and validating the skills and abilities of staff members to ensure that they meet the organization's standards. If the quality of staff skills and abilities remains high, then it is likely that the quality of patient care and services will also remain high. This chapter defines key competency-related terms and explains the various ways in which healthcare organizations apply the term "competency assessment."

What is competency?

Competency is the demonstrated ability to fulfill the primary responsibilities of the position for which a person was hired. Observing and measuring competency for every position in the facility, including health-occupation students (i.e., students of nursing, pharmacy, imaging, and rehabilitation, etc.) and volunteers who work in the same capacity as staff in providing care, treatment, or service, gives leaders confidence that healthcare providers are exercising care, caution, and concern for the patients.

Why develop a competency program?

Healthcare facilities should develop competency programs for several reasons, one of which is that TJC requires such programs. However, competency programs are important for reasons other than TJC compliance. Well-designed competency programs have three important functions:

- To help facility leaders stay focused on their primary objective: the facility's mission statement

- To assist in matching applicants to open positions

Chapter One

- To ensure ongoing assessment of staff competency from system entry through the remainder of the person's association with the organization

The following TJC HR standards provide the framework for a comprehensive competency program. They also guide HR department personnel and department leaders in developing a program that fulfills the above three functions and supports their expectations of performance in the facility and their departments:

- HR.1 requires leaders to identify the qualifications for each position in the facility, addresses at-hire competency validation, and requires leaders to ensure staffing effectiveness.

- HR.2 requires facilities to orient new staff, students, and volunteers to the organization, the department/unit/area in which they will work, and their job; establishes a process to validate staff, student, and volunteer competency by the end of orientation; and provides continuing education and training.

- HR.3 requires leaders to establish a process for validating ongoing competency of staff, students, and volunteers who work in the same capacity as staff providing care, treatment, or service; and to periodically conduct staff performance reviews.

Developing a specific goal with clearly defined objectives will assist leaders in implementing a meaningful competency assessment program. Below is a sample goal for a competency assessment program:

The goal of the competency assessment program is to fulfill the mission, vision, and value statements of the hospital by ensuring that qualified and competent staff provide high-quality services.

Objectives of the competency program are to:

- Establish a policy that defines the competency program on the facilitywide and department-specific levels

- Develop and implement the following department-specific components:

    - Competency-based job descriptions for every position in every department
    - Orientation programs for every department/unit that includes the department's functions and responsibilities

- Develop each leader's interview and critical judgment skills in order to enable him or her to identify those candidates who will successfully fill open positions

- Establish a background check that includes:

    - A completed application

    - Primary source verification and validation of licensure, certification, or registration, when required by law in order to practice

    - Verification and validation of licensure, certification, or registration, when required by the organization

    - Reference checks of personal and professional contacts

    - Criminal and other background checks as required by the organization

- Establish a mechanism to ensure that every employee attends all aspects of orientation required by the organization for completion by clinical staff before the individual begins providing care, treatment, or service to patients; attends the aspects of orientation to the job for which the organization has determined the employee can be oriented as he or she provides care, treatment, or service; and orientation to the facility within the time defined by organization leaders

- Establish a plan to ensure that competency is validated within the designated orientation period

- Ensure that performance evaluations are completed and given to the employee in the time frame established in the facility's policy

- Participate in an ongoing educational program and a competency validation process that are based in part on the results of performance evaluations and other data sources

- Design department-specific educational programs that target improvement in staff competency

- Establish a database to ensure that licenses, certifications, and registrations are current

CHAPTER ONE

Who needs to be assessed?

All staff members—including those providing care, treatment, or service under contractual arrangements—students, and volunteers who work in the same capacity as staff providing care, treatment, or service need to be assessed. Every employee in the facility is responsible for certain duties, and each employee must be able to perform his or her duties competently. Every employee should also be familiar with the policies and procedures relevant to his or her duties and know how those duties contribute to quality patient care, treatment, and service, and how they support the functioning of his or her department.

Department leaders should ensure that each employee understands the expectations/responsibilities/activities/competencies required for his or her position. Armed with this information, each employee will better understand his or her department leader's expectations regarding qualified and knowledgeable staff.

Who conducts competency assessments?

The department leader ensures the completion of competency assessments in one of four ways. He or she does one of the following:

- Designates a person who is responsible for all new-hire orientation and competency validation

- Establishes a proctoring system in which qualified personnel perform competency verification at the time of orientation and on an ongoing basis thereafter

- Obtains competency-related information from a combination of input from supervisors and direct observation

- Chooses to perform all competency assessments for all employees himself or herself

It's important to remember that the person validating someone else's competency must be qualified to do so. For example, if the pharmacy director isn't a pharmacist, he or she cannot validate the clinical competency of the pharmacist working in the department. Another example involves the director of a home care program validating clinical competency of all staff, including the clinical staff in rehabilitation, nutrition, etc. Since the director is likely not clinically competent in all these disciplines, he or she is not qualified to validate clinical competency of staff. In either example, the director can complete the staff's performance reviews, but he or she cannot validate their clinical competency. We will discuss this idea more in Chapter 3.

Who determines which competencies need to be assessed, and how are those competencies chosen?

The leaders of the organization determine which competencies must be assessed. This responsibility includes initial competencies, competencies to be assessed (i.e., validated) by the end of orientation, and those to be assessed (i.e., validated) on an ongoing basis.

Initial competency must be met in order for the individual to join the organization. This is sometimes known as at-hire competency validation. It is a process a representative from the human resources department and the unit/department leader often share. It involves verifying whether the prospective employee or volunteer meets the qualifications specified in the job description/position description. It includes verifying his or her licensure, registration, certification, education, and any other requirements specified. It is the role of leaders to identify the qualifications needed for each position in the organization. If the job is one in which care, treatment, or service is provided to patients, the qualifications should be identified after considering the patient populations to whom this care, treatment, or service is to be provided.

It is also the role of leaders to identify the responsibilities or activities the individual will be expected to perform. These responsibilities can also be thought of as competencies. They are identified in the job description/position description as primary responsibilities. The individual must prove competent to perform each of the primary responsibilities by the end of the orientation period. Because these are primary responsibilities of the position, they are likely to be performed with some degree of regularity by all staff members in the job group or all staff members having the same job title, i.e., all respiratory therapists, all cashiers, etc. As such, they represent "core competencies" or "core responsibilities." Some staff members in the job group may have additional responsibilities because of the unit/department in which they work or the patient population for whom they provide care, treatment, or service.

Following the orientation period, the individual begins to perform his or her job without supervision, moving into ongoing competency validation. Figure 1.1 includes definitions and examples of low-volume/high-risk, changed or new, mandated by a regulatory agency or by the organization as requiring annual education and revalidation of competency, and problem-prone responsibilities that could be identified as ongoing competencies for various staff situations.

Chapter One

> **Figure 1.1: Definitions and examples of low-volume/high-risk, new or changed, problem-prone, and mandated duties**
>
> Low-volume/high-risk duties are rarely performed duties that carry a significant risk of hazard or harm. Examples of such duties include a respiratory therapist stabilizing a premature infant for transport to a tertiary care neonatal intensive care unit, a nurse assisting with the insertion of a chest tube on a medical-surgical unit, and a staff member monitoring a patient receiving sedation for an invasive procedure.
>
> New duties are responsibilities that will be performed for the first time, and changed activities are those that are planned to be performed in a different way. Examples include the use by respiratory therapists of newly purchased ventilators, the introduction of physician computerized order entry, and bar coding for medication administration.
>
> Problem-prone duties are frequently or infrequently performed duties for which some data source has indicated a problem in performance. Examples include staff response to a fire drill, performance of CPR, administration of medications, collection of blood specimens for testing, and staff response to a faulty generator switch during generator testing.
>
> Activities/responsibilities mandated for ongoing competency may be frequently or infrequently performed duties that an external regulatory agency, the organization itself, or the unit/department in which the individual works has mandated to be assessed for ongoing competency on an annual basis. Examples include waived testing proficiency, and restraint usage.

When do employees need their competencies assessed?

Note: Chapter 4 discusses the competency assessment cycle in more detail.
The organization must assess every employee's competency:

- Before the employee is hired (initial competency assessment)

- During orientation (validation primary responsibilities/activities can be performed satisfactorily)

- On an ongoing basis after orientation (ongoing competency assessment)

Initial competency assessment

This review helps eliminate candidates who do not have the necessary education, training, or experience for the open position. Through this process of elimination, the department leader avoids wasting time interviewing unqualified candidates. Once the applicants' qualifications are verified, the unit/department leader then interviews the remaining applicants, confirming each applicant's work experience and exploring his or her knowledge base.

A critical component of initial competency verification is "primary source verification" of the individual's current license, registration, or certification when this document is required by law to practice in that job title. Often the requirement is found in a practice act, such as the practice act issued by a state board of pharmacy, or by a board of nursing.

The concept and process for primary source verification is one in which staff members in the medical staff office are well versed, but it is still relatively new for staff outside this area. The requirement for primary source verification of a nonphysician license, registration, or certification was extended by TJC to nonphysician staff within the last few years, and still leaves some organizations struggling to understand the expectations and design a process to ensure not only that the individual possesses a current and valid license, registration, or certificate prior to employment, but also that he or she renews the license, certificate, or registration prior to its expiration. It is important to stress that this is not a concept applied only to RNs. All staff members for whom the license, certificate, or registration is required by law in order to practice must be part of the identified process for primary source verification.

Examples of nonphysician staff members for whom a license, registration, or certification is required in order to practice include the registered nurse, licensed practical nurse, certified nursing assistant, pharmacist, dietitian, respiratory therapist, rehabilitation professional (PT/OT/SLP), and social worker. With primary source verification, the agency/board issuing the document is contacted to verify that the individual received the document in question. In many situations this can be done electronically between you and the agency.

Leaders must define a process to verify any license, registration, or certification required by the organization but not required by law in order to practice. In this situation, the organization must identify, by job title, all licensure, certification, or registrations it requires of staff members in certain job groups/job titles and to determine the process for verifying that the individual possesses the required certificate, license, or registration. It is up to the organization to determine the process it will follow for this verification.

An example might be the organization that requires all respiratory therapists (RTs) to maintain current certification in basic life support (BLS). The process for verifying this certification should, at a minimum, include viewing the original document issued to the individual.

An additional consideration of leaders is the process to use in verifying any education required for the position. Options include primary source verification of education, prior to or during the interview process. In this scenario, the school(s) the individual attended would be contacted and asked to verify that the individual graduated. The alternative to primary source verification is to request to view the originals of all these documents. Many organizations simply accept the job applicant's documentation that the applicant attained the required education. Licensure, registration, or certification cannot be obtained in the absence of clinical education.

Validation of core competency by the end of orientation

Verification that the primary responsibilities of the job can be performed according to unit/department standards occurs during the individual's orientation to his or her unit/department and job. This ensures a consistent level of performance by all individuals in the same job group or having the same job title, regardless of the unit/department to which they are assigned. Before being assigned to tasks and duties, the new employee must be prepared to perform them in accordance with the organization's policies and procedures. Orientation serves to educate the individual on unit/department expectations, train the individual in the accepted way to perform the primary/essential responsibilities of the job, and allows the individual to demonstrate his or her ability to competently perform the primary responsibilities of the job for which he or she was hired.

The identification of primary activities/responsibilities expected of staff in any job title/job group begins by identifying those activities/responsibilities expected of all staff in a job group (e.g., all RNs, all pharmacists, all registrars, all security officers, all insurance verifiers, etc.). Because these activities/responsibilities are expected of all staff, they can be thought of as core responsibilities/activities. For many employees, this represents the entirety of their job responsibilities/activities. For others, there are additional responsibilities/activities expected of all staff in a job group/job title, employed in a specific unit/area/department of the organization, in addition to those activities/

responsibilities already identified as core competencies. These activities are reflective of the additional patient populations, activities, or technology found only in these sites. Examples include an RN in an oncology unit administering chemotherapy, and a pharmacist in the hospital's outpatient dispensing pharmacy responsible for enrolling patients in the community's medication purchase assistance program.

For those staff members in clinical positions providing care, treatment, or service to patients, there is an additional consideration—patient age or patient population. If the patients are of different age groups or different populations that requires their care, treatment, or service be altered in some way when it is provided to them, then it is a competency with an age-related or a population-related aspect to it. Assessing a staff member's ability to competently perform a responsibility with an age-related or population-related aspect means the staff member's ability to appropriately alter the way he or she carries out the responsibility must be validated. This is done at the same time the competency itself is validated, and will be discussed more in Chapter 2.

An example of an activity with an age-related aspect is taking vital signs, because the healthcare provider must select a different size cuff for taking blood pressure based on patients' ages, use different methods to take a temperature in different age groups, and know the different ranges that qualify as normal for various age groups for all vital signs taken.

CHAPTER ONE

> **TJC switch from age-related to population-related care**
>
> For all the frenzy associated with the need to demonstrate "age-appropriate care" delivery ("care appropriate to the needs of the populations served" in the 2004 standards), it is only referenced twice in the standards. It's found in the standards directing the organization to consider the patient age groups served (populations served after 2004) when planning or sponsoring staff attendance during ongoing training or continuing education programs. The other is in the standards related to leaders considering the ages of the patients (patient populations after 2004) to whom care is provided when determining the qualifications for particular jobs and again when directing leaders to periodically evaluate/assess/validate staff competency to provide patient care. Does this mean the need to demonstrate age-appropriate care has been eliminated? No. Patient age groups can represent patient populations. But, in addition, there are other ways to get staff to identify a group of patients whose care must be altered in some way to meet their unique needs. Examples of other ways to cohort patients (i.e., patient populations) include situations such as the patient with sensory impairments if providing patient education, the bariatric patient when positioning for operative and invasive procedures, the patient at the end of life when managing pain, etc. Recognizing patient age groups as populations is as relevant today as it ever was, but it is not the only way to cohort patients with unique needs.

Ongoing competency assessment

The ongoing competency assessment consists of selected skills, duties, or tasks performed in the department that the unit/department leader has determined to be important enough to measure and evaluate throughout the year. Ongoing competency assessments ensure that staff have improved or maintained skills in the important areas under review. Unlike competency validation at the end of orientation, the ongoing competency assessment is not comprehensive. Ongoing competency assessments entail a short list chosen from analysis of available data such as the results of performance-improvement activities, infection-control reviews, and risk-management reviews, additions of new technology or changes to existing processes, those competencies mandated by an external regulatory agency as needing annual reeducation and competency validation, and responsibilities occurring infrequently. Some of the responsibilities on the list will appear year after year, while others, such as those that are new or changed, are only identified for a particular year. The list of competencies chosen for any year is small. After choosing the ongoing competencies, the unit/department leader develops guidelines for evaluating and measuring each competency. If an activity on the ongoing competency list is one that has already been identified as having an age or population-related aspect to it (see previous sidebar), then it is a given that the activity continues to have this age or population-related aspect to it each time it is validated. Below is a representation of the thought process inherent in the identification of ongoing competencies. It represents the four questions applied to the primary responsibilities/activities/competencies of any job, and is to be asked for both the core responsibilities and the additional responsibilities for all staff members.

Ongoing competence decision tree

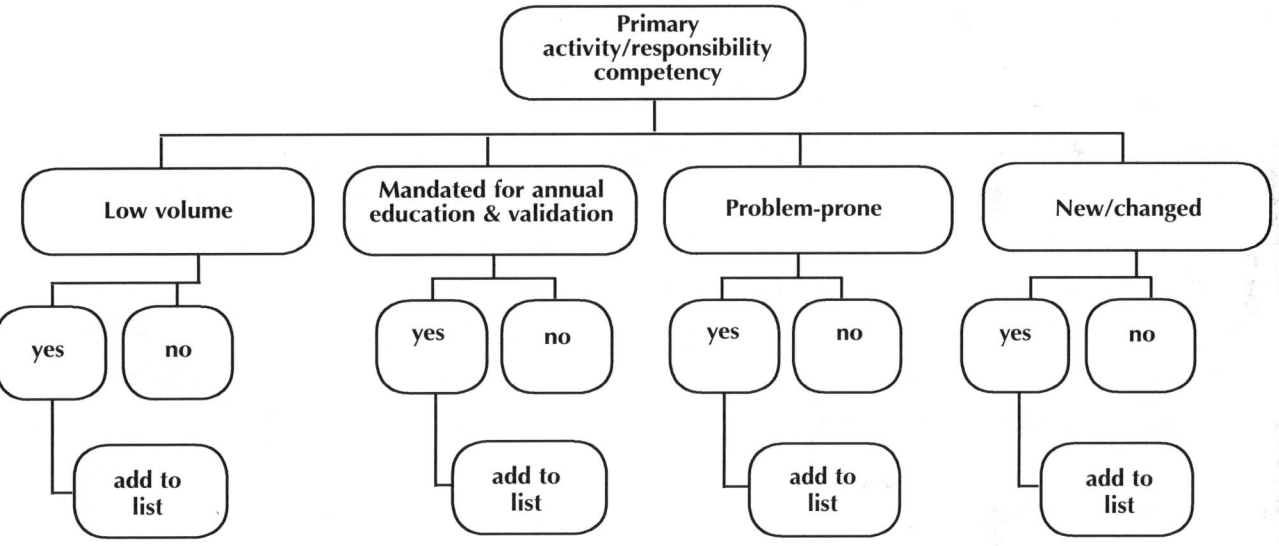

The process of identifying the activities/responsibilities/competencies for ongoing (i.e., annual) education and validation of competency is not something to be done only once. An analogous process in healthcare is the budget cycle. No organization casts a budget only once. It is an annual process, with monthly analysis of data in order to spot variances, so that action might be taken to return to the budgeted parameters. The same concept applies to that of ongoing competency.

Leaders project the activities/responsibilities/competencies for the coming year for which staff members will be provided education and then have competency validated. They then monitor the available data for signs of variance that require unplanned action. In the case of ongoing competency, this means adding activities/responsibilities/competencies to the existing list and providing staff with education, then validating/revalidating competency.

Chapter One

Deciding which activities/responsibilities/competencies from the entire list of activities/responsibilities/competencies must be addressed through ongoing competency validation must be specific to the job itself. The questions that determine the composition of the list must be asked first of all staff in a job title (core expectations of all staff in a job group) and then the same questions asked for staff having additional responsibilities beyond core.

Just as with core competencies, some ongoing competencies could have an age- or population-related aspect to them, so competency assessment must include an assessment of the person's ability to appropriately alter the care, treatment, or service he or she performs, when this is needed.

Here are two examples that should serve to clarify these concepts. For the first example, let's use an RT. One of the primary activities/responsibilities/competencies of an RT is that of medication administration via the inhalation route. Competency to perform this activity would begin during orientation. The new employee would receive education about how this is to be done at the organization at which he or she is working and then have his or her competency validated to perform this activity. In the case of medication administration, competency validation should reflect the individual's ability to alter the performance of the task as appropriate to the age of the patient. Once this competency is validated, this activity is one the individual respiratory therapist is likely to perform regularly. Unless a problem is identified through a review of the data or the process to follow in providing this care to patients is planned to change in the immediate future, the individual demonstrates ongoing competency in this core responsibility each day he or she works. If this were not the case, some data source would reveal a problem in the performance of the activity.

For the second example, let's use an RN. The orientation for an RN includes a comprehensive review of the organization's expectations (i.e., policy and tools for assessing pain) regarding a comprehensive pain assessment. All newly hired RNs would be required to attend orientation and complete the competency validation. This would not be expected of staff members who do not have pain assessment listed as a primary job responsibility. During the year, the organization collects pain-assessment data through performance improvement monitoring activities, patient perception surveys, complaint logs, etc. Leaders use these data to identify the ongoing competency of staff. In our example, let's pretend the data show that two areas of pain assessment are not in compliance with the targeted indicators. Leaders include these two indicators on the list of ongoing competencies to be assessed/validated for the year. In this process, leaders utilize the performance improvement resource to identify areas in which the employees are no longer demonstrating continued competency, as well as to identify the areas in which they do continue to demonstrate competency. Since the tools to use in assessing pain for patients of different ages should differ, this also represents an activity/responsibility with an age-specific aspect to the process.

Chapter Two

Competency assessments and the Joint Commission standards

Competency assessments and the Joint Commission standards

Introduction

The Joint Commission (TJC) requires all healthcare organizations to provide a sufficient number of qualified and competent staff to meet the needs of their patients and it requires each organization to provide staff members with opportunities to maintain and improve competency. Organization leaders must ensure there is validation of staff competency at hire, by the end of orientation, and on an ongoing basis. The Joint Commission's competency standards are challenging to many healthcare settings and have historically been among the most often-cited recommendations.

This chapter examines TJC's competency requirements in detail. It explains surveyor expectations, discusses relevant issues and hot buttons, and suggests practical strategies for compliance. Although the focus of this book is on competency and TJC standards, we would be remiss if we did not briefly discuss the other requirements found in the HR standards.

The Joint Commission requirements for competency, education, and periodic performance reviews apply to all employees in every setting, including those employees who never have direct patient contact. It is important to note that the requirements also apply to staff members who provide care, treatment, and service under contractual arrangements; to students; and to volunteers serving in the same capacity as staff in providing care, treatment, or service. The competency standards are generally the same for all healthcare settings. Figure 2.1, at the end of the chapter, provides a competency assessment tool to help you ensure that the various steps in the process have been followed.

Defining job qualifications and providing qualified staff

Defining qualifications
It is the role of organizational leaders to define the qualifications for the various jobs

Chapter Two

performed within the organization and to ensure there is a process in place to verify that prospective employees meet the stated qualifications prior to employment.

Initial competency validation, or at-hire competency validation, can be thought of as the process of ensuring that someone is qualified to enter the work site. Only those individuals who meet the required qualifications should be allowed to work in the organization, regardless of whether they are attempting to work as employees of the organization, as contracted or agency personnel, or as volunteers if they serve in the same capacity as staff providing care, treatment, or service.

Organizations should validate competency for all applicants before they start work. HR.1 requires that facilities screen each applicant to ensure that he or she meets the qualifications stated in the job description. These qualifications include:

- Education
- Licensure
- Registration
- Certification
- Experience
- Health screening
- Criminal background check

Although we often think about these qualifications in terms of clinical staff, organizations should state these qualifications in all job descriptions and verify each applicant's qualifications before hire. For example, an employee in the hospital's transportation department might be required to have a current driver's license, and a plumber might be required to have a current plumber's license or certificate.

The department leader should determine the qualifications for each position after reviewing the essential responsibilities of the job and the patient age groups and populations to which the employee will be expected to provide care, treatment, or service, if applicable. For example, the responsibility of individual and group counseling of adolescents might require a master's degree in social work or psychology with a year's experience counseling adolescents, while the responsibilities of counseling an adult population might require the individual to have a license in clinical social work (LCSW).

Because it has thoughtfully identified the required qualifications for each position, an organization should not ignore those qualifications, regardless of how badly it needs staff. In addition to the potential of receiving a recommendation from TJC, failure to completely validate an employee's competency before he or she begins to deliver care could negatively affect patient care.

What do TJC surveyors expect?

TJC surveyors expect each facility to do the following:

- Define qualifications for every position. To define qualifications, review the patient populations to which the employee would be expected to deliver care or service, the essential responsibilities of the job, and any anticipated changes in the job that might require new or current employees to possess additional qualifications.

- Complete the first phase of competency validation by verifying that applicants possess all required qualifications before hire. Complete this verification for all employed staff members, contract staff members, and volunteers. Typically, HR staff members complete this phase, then share their findings with the department manager so that he or she can decide whether to proceed with interviewing and possibly hiring the applicant.

    See Chapter 1 for more about primary source verification.

- Maintain records of all verified qualifications, including the dates on which they were verified and the names of staff members who completed the verifications. Organizations usually maintain these records in employees' HR files, but they may maintain them in any other place they deem suitable.

- Include all staff in the competency assessment program.

Relevant issues

Ensuring an adequate number of qualified staff members remains one of the most difficult tasks for today's healthcare leaders. There are highly publicized shortages of various healthcare workers in almost every area of the country. Recruitment and retention efforts have taken on a new importance. When efforts to recruit staff fail, many organizations turn to staffing agencies for relief. The more critical the need, the more tempting it becomes to hire the individual before completing competency validation. This strategy will only prove costly in the long run.

Compliance tips

Avoiding TJC citations in the area of competency assessment begins with the job description itself, which should clearly delineate the qualifications for the job. These qualifications should reflect organizational analysis of the services the facility offers and the populations it serves. Unless there is a compelling reason to do otherwise, applicants should not be hired unless they fully meet the qualifications. A compelling example of when to overlook specific qualifications might be if a potential hire has an advanced educational degree and only 18 months of experience, which may outweigh the requirement for three years of experience. Such situations should be the exception, not the rule, and this decision-making process should be reflected in the employee's personnel file in case of questions about initial competency validation. Likewise, those providing care or service under contractual arrangements should meet the same qualifications as those individuals hired by the organization.

The job description should also identify the ages of patients to whom the individual will be expected to provide care or service, as surveyors will expect the competency validation tools to include this information. Organizations should ensure that there is organizationwide agreement as to what these age groups are and the definition of each. Without this uniformity, competency validation—particularly cross-training among disciplines and between departments—becomes difficult.

Staffing

Staffing adequacy

It is also an organization's leaders' responsibility to determine the number of staff members needed to provide care, treatment, and service to patients. They then have to ensure that a sufficient array of qualified and competent staff members—both in terms of numbers of staff members and skill mix of staff members—are present to meet the needs of patients. This is known as staffing adequacy. The assessment of staffing adequacy is subjective (it's currently a "B" element of performance), and is rarely an issue at the time of survey. If a surveyor had concerns, he or she would ask for comparison data between the number and skill mix of staff members working over a period of time to the number and skill mix required in the organization's staffing plan.

Staffing effectiveness

Several years ago, TJC added to its expectations for staffing adequacy by calling for an assessment of staffing effectiveness. The focus today is on nurse staffing and nursing-sensitive outcome indicators, and will likely remain so in the future. This is a departure from the original standards in effect for the first few years, in which other disciplines were also included in the human resource–indicator data collection and analysis.

The change, which was effective in July 2005, places the focus of staffing effectiveness analysis clearly on nurse staffing. It requires all levels of nursing (i.e., RN, LPN, nursing assistants/aides) to be included in the human resource data collection and analysis. It does not require other nonnursing staff members to be included in the analysis, but this is permissible if the organization chooses to do so.

The change reduced the units' populations/settings for which data must be gathered to two inpatient units, rather than selecting indicators that address all patient populations in an organization. It required the selection of two indicator sets (one clinical and one HR indicator) for each unit. The list of outcome indicators provided by TJC from which the organization must choose includes clinical indicators thought to be sensitive to nurse staffing and represents work already done by the National Quality Forum (NQF) nursing-sensitive patient care measures. Many organizations already routinely collect and analyze data for many of the NQF clinical indicators. The standards require leaders to consider a host of factors when identifying the indicators for data collection and analysis.

Another important change in the standards is that there is no expectation that the organization will look for statistical correlation when analyzing its data, but it will look for possible relationships between the indicators. In other words, the expectation that the indicators be analyzed in relation to each other is eliminated. In truth, this was never meant to be a research project where the organization collected data in order to prove or disprove a hypothesis, though it fell just short of this in some organizations.

In brief, here are the steps to the staffing effectiveness standards:

- Select at least two inpatient units/departments for which data will be gathered
- Select two indicator sets, using the criteria specified, to include input from the staff
- Standardize definitions for each indicator
- Determine thresholds for each indicator
- Collect and analyze data for all indicators
- Drill down when thresholds are exceeded for any indicator when compared to its threshold
- Review data for indicator sets, looking for possible relationships
- Take action as appropriate
- Report to leadership annually

The underlying principle is that only by looking at the relationship between human resource indicators and clinical/service outcome indicators can decisions about staffing effectiveness be made.

Clinical/service indicators are such things as patient falls, medication errors, and customer satisfaction. Examples of human resource indicators are such things as vacancy rates, hours per patient day, and overtime hours. The Joint Commission has included in the HR standards a list of both types of indicators. Leaders are to select at least two indicator sets (one set of clinical/service indicators and one set of human resource indicators in each indicator set, for a total of four indicators) and gather data about each in order to determine whether a relationship exists between any of them. If a relationship is seen, TJC expects action at the leadership level. Most organizations have seen little or no relationship between the human resource indicators and the clinical/service indicators selected for analysis, but it remains a worthwhile endeavor nevertheless.

Disaster responsibilities

The opportunity to use nonphysician health providers, such as RNs, pharmacists, imaging staff, rehabilitation staff, social workers, etc., in emergency situations (e.g., Hurricane Katrina) was added to the HR standards in 2006. HR.1.25 has the same wording as the standard for physician volunteers that had been a part of TJC's standards for several years prior to this. The decision to accept nonphysician volunteers to provide assistance in a disaster is one the leaders must address in policy. If the decision is that volunteers will not be accepted to help staff an emergency, the policy is a statement to this effect and nothing more need be done. If, however, the decision is that volunteers will be accepted, a process to accept volunteers, including the primary source verification of any license, registration, or certification required by law to practice, must be a part of the identified process.

The qualification, orientation, and competency of physician-employed staff members brought into the healthcare setting are also addressed in the HR standards (i.e., physician-employed office nurse or private scrub). The expectation is that the qualifications and competency of these individuals must be reviewed by the organization's leaders and found to be commensurate to that of hospital-employed staff, and that the hospital reviews the qualification, performance, and competency of each individual with the same frequency as for hospital-employed staff.

Note that this standard is not focused on physician assistants or nurse practitioners. The qualifications, responsibilities, and competency of these individuals are also found in the HR standards, but actually follow a different standard than the one addressing physician-employed non-advanced-practice staff. The qualifications, responsibilities, and competency of these individuals are usually addressed through the process used for the medical staff, and are not the focus of the physician-employed non-advanced-practice staff.

Orientation, education, and training of staff members

Orientation

Orientation is actually a form of staff training and education, as is attending a seminar or a workshop, a professional association education program, or a myriad of other educational offerings to continue staff development. Orientation is designated as education for new employees. All employees, students, and volunteers should be required to complete orientation and have competency validated at the end of orientation. In addition, forensic staff—law enforcement officers who accompany a prisoner to the hospital and stay with their prisoner, now your patient, for the entire time the prisoner receives care at the hospital—must be oriented to certain prescribed activities of concern to them and the organization.

Although the organization may include additional items if it wishes, TJC standards require the following items be addressed in orientation for forensic staff:

- The difference between administrative and clinical restraint
- Channels of administrative, security, and clinical communication that officers should follow
- How to interact with patients (e.g., patient privacy and confidentiality, etc.)
- What officers should do if there is an unusual clinical event or incident (e.g., if a patient suffers cardiac arrest)

For students, volunteers, and those who provide care or service under contractual arrangements, this orientation is often abbreviated but must always include the requirements for general safety, fire safety, infection control, and the Health Insurance Portability and Accountability Act as well as orientation to the work environment and to their specific responsibilities.

Orientation serves many functions. It introduces new employees to the organization and to their roles. New employees learn what is acceptable and what is not acceptable. They learn about their jobs, organizational and departmental procedures, equipment they will routinely use in performing their jobs, and their roles in ensuring a safe work environment for themselves and others.

Orientation to the organization should include information about the following:

- The organization's mission and goals
- Cultural diversity and sensitivity (to staff and patients)
- Patient rights
- Ethical issues and how to respond to them
- Roles and responsibilities in patient safety and in environmental safety
- How to recognize and respond to unusual occurrences
- How to recognize and minimize risks employees may encounter within the organization

Interacting with your patient (the prisoner of the forensic officer) while in your facility might require some different behaviors on the part of forensic staff members than those they exhibit within their usual work environment. If so, they need to know what your expectations are. One area that needs to be clarified early on involves the use of administrative restraint and response to clinical emergencies. There must be a clear understanding that if a forensic staff member is asked to remove the administrative restraint to allow care to be provided to the patient, this must occur without hesitation on their part.

Following orientation to the organization, individuals must be oriented to the unit/department in which they will work. It is here that the organizational information is individualized to the unique expectations of staff in that unit/department. For example, at orientation to the organization, the staff is educated about the organization's fire response process and its role in a fire, whether staff members find the fire or respond to the announcement that a fire has been detected. Orientation to the unit/department educates the individual as to the location of fire extinguishers and the fire alarms in that particular setting. The egress routes to be used by that unit/department staff, if needed, are reviewed. Any additional fire-response supplies or equipment unique to that unit/department also are identified, and staff members are educated on how to use them.

The individual also must be oriented to the specific job for which he or she was hired or to the specific activities he or she will be performing as a volunteer. It is during orientation that managers evaluate employees' abilities to carry out the essential functions of their jobs. If a job involves regular clinical contact with patients, and the same function must be performed differently for patients of different ages or different populations, the manager must assess the employee's ability to deliver care appropriately to patients of different ages or populations. Such an assessment is commonly referred to as age-appropriate/age-specific or population-appropriate/population-specific competency validation.

Determining which employees have regular clinical contact with patients is not as obvious as it might seem. Some staff members clearly have no patient contact at all—for example, staff members in the finance, medical records, and information services departments. Other staff members clearly do have regular patient contact. Examples include nursing and respiratory therapy.

However, there are some employees for whom this determination is less obvious, such as security and environmental services staff members. For example, many organizations require security officers to respond to violent and aggressive patient/visitor situations. Security officers often participate in "take down," clinical "holds," and restraints. Participating in these clinical activities is defined as employees having regular, but specific, clinical contact with patients. Because holds and restraints should be applied differently to patients of different ages, these activities qualify as age-specific clinical tasks. Competency validation for these tasks should include assessment of how staff would modify or change the performance of these tasks based on patients' ages.

Managers must decide whether staff members have regular clinical contact with patients only after reviewing their job descriptions and reviewing how they were oriented to their jobs. Well-written job descriptions should help determine which staff members have regular clinical contact with patients and whether the organization must validate their abilities to deliver care or service in a manner appropriate to the patient's age. See Chapter 5 for a discussion about validating competencies with an age-related aspect to them.

Compliance tips
The following are some tips to comply with the competency assessment standards:

- Provide all new employees, students, and volunteers with a proper orientation. An employee's competency begins with the orientation process, which determines his or her capacity to perform job responsibilities.

- Make sure the orientation process provides initial job training and information.

- Be sure to conduct orientation for contract/agency staff members and for forensic staff members. They need to know what to do in case of a fire, how to protect patient rights, and how to maintain patient confidentiality.

- Document attendance at completion of the orientation program in each employee's personnel record.

- Orientation is designed to promote safe and effective performance. Therefore, organizations should use orientation to familiarize staff members with their responsibilities and/or work environments before initiating patient care and other activities.

Ongoing education

In addition to providing orientation, organizations must provide ongoing education—such as inservice programs, attendance at seminars, articles for review, brown-bag discussion groups, and other activities—to maintain and improve staff competency. Continuing education should occur whenever the job duties change, when a learning need has been identified through a review of available data, and in situations in which an external regulatory agency mandates education be provided. Education should address the needs of the various patient age groups and populations to whom care, treatment, or service is provided. Information on team training should be provided whenever it is determined to be needed. A completed root-cause analysis (RCA) following a sentinel event or a completed failure modes and effects analysis (FMEA) acts as a vehicle to identify the need for team training.

What do TJC surveyors expect?

TJC surveyors examine personnel files for evidence that the organization verified each employee's education, training, and appropriate knowledge and experience.

Relevant issues

Orientation is the organization's first opportunity to offer staff education and training. All training and education is intended to either maintain or improve staff competency, but education is not competency validation. Those who provide the educational or training program must include an activity to validate that staff members who attend the program have mastered the material presented and can reflect this reinforced or new knowledge in performing their jobs. Orientation carries the same expectation of competency validation as all other training and education.

In fact, it is at the end of the orientation period—the organization should define the length of this period—that the organization verifies the employee's competency to perform the essential responsibilities of his or her job. This is the second point in the competency validation cycle. Please see Chapter 4 for a complete discussion of the competency validation cycle.

Compliance tips

- Education and training programs should improve employee knowledge of specific work-related issues. Organizations should periodically review staff members' abilities to carry out job responsibilities, especially when introducing new procedures, techniques, technologies, and/or equipment.

- It is important to remember that TJC requires organizations to educate staff members about the role of the environment of care in safety and patient care. In each of the seven management plans required in the Environment of Care (EC) standards—safety, security, hazardous materials and waste, emergency preparedness, life safety, medical equipment, and utility systems—TJC requires organizations to orient and educate staff.

Assessing staff members' competency

Competency validation at end of orientation

Competency must be validated at the end of the orientation period. This allows the unit/department leader to determine whether the individual is competent to carry out the primary functions or responsibilities of his or her job.

Ongoing competency

Once employees complete orientation and validate core and additional (if indicated) competencies (the ability to carry out the primary responsibilities of their job), organizations must validate ongoing competency. Such assessments should reflect the changing nature of the job, any responsibilities occurring infrequently (low-volume activities), any aspects of the job expected to change in the coming year, and any problem-prone aspects of the job that have been identified through review of existing data. Chapter 3 addresses the data sources that can be used both as a measure of ongoing competency and as a source of identifying learning needs with concomitant competency validation following the education.

The ongoing competencies identified for validation will reflect some similarities to those validated by the end of orientation, but should reflect differences, as well. Any responsibility/activity/competency identified for ongoing competency that has an age-related or population-related aspect to its performance must have this aspect of competency validated, much as it was for competency validation at the end of orientation.

Chapter Two

What do TJC surveyors expect?
Surveyors determine whether you have periodically assessed, as appropriate, an employee's ability to provide care for the age groups or populations specified in the job description.

Sentinel events and competency assessments

Sentinel event literature is focusing more attention on the HR standards. These include the standards that relate to adequacy of staffing, communication, and team dynamics and the need to ensure that a facility has a competent staff, including those providing care, treatment, or service under a contractual arrangement. Analysis of reported sentinel events indicates these areas to be the top three most frequently cited contributing causes of all sentinel events reported to the Joint Commission.

Compliance tips
Organizations may choose from a variety of tools for competency validation and performance review. Organizations should select tools based on ease of use and the job duties for which the individual is responsible. Chapter 7 includes examples from a number of different settings and may prove helpful in designing a process for your organization.

Particularly with competency validation and performance review, "packaging"—how the tools look and how they are displayed—is sometimes as important as what the tools contain. If surveyors cannot identify an individual's job responsibilities, cannot find evidence of age-specific or populator specific competency consistent with the ages or populations identified in the job description, or cannot find an apparent methodology for competency validation, the organization will be at risk for a requirement for improvement.

Performance evaluation
While competency validation ensures the individual can fulfill the primary responsibilities of his or her job, performance evaluations ensure the individual continues to meet the "citizenship" obligations of the job. This includes such things as maintaining licensure, registration, or certification; attendance at required continuing-education programs; compliance with the dress code; support of corporate mission and values; customer satisfaction; use of personal protective equipment (PPE); participation in performance improvement activities; etc. Performance expectations can be thought of as "organizational citizenship" expectations. While the performance evaluation findings and the summary review

of ongoing competency may occur at the same time, they are addressing two different aspects of the individual's activities. Organizations strive to attract and retain competent staff members who are also good corporate citizens. Both expectations must be assessed at a frequency identified by the organization.

Organizations must define the frequency with which performance is evaluated. The time between evaluations cannot exceed three years. Most organizations complete performance evaluations annually.

How often does an organization have to validate competency?
The organization must validate the competency of all staff; including those providing care under contractual arrangements; students; and volunteers serving in the same capacity as staff in providing care, treatment, or service:

- at hire
- at the end of the orientation period
- on an ongoing basis following orientation

In addition, the organization must complete periodic performance evaluations for all staff members. Although competency validation occurs throughout the year, the formal review with the employee is often held once each year, often at the same time as his or her performance review. Please see Chapter 4 for a discussion of the competency validation cycle and Chapter 5 for a discussion of ways to verify competency.

How does TJC survey competency assessment?
The surveyors will take note of staff members with whom they interact while conducting tracer activities, and will ask to see their orientation and competency validation materials. This request may come during the actual tracer, with the process halting as the surveyor reviews the materials provided, or the surveyor may request the materials during tracer activity but review them at the end of the day. Sometimes all or a portion of the review of materials is completed during the competency validation session—it is up to the survey team. Whatever way is used, when the surveyor asks for the orientation and competency validation materials for a particular staff member or volunteer, it is incumbent upon the organization to quickly and easily assemble the requested materials, regardless of where they are normally located. This expectation includes any materials requested for agency/contract staff.

Chapter Two

Surveyors review the following data in each employee's file:

- Job description

- Primary source verification of initial and current licensure/registration/certification

- Completion of orientation to the hospital, to his or her work area, and to his or her specific job duties

- Competency validation by the end of orientation and ongoing competency validation, as appropriate to length of service, including the ability to provide age-appropriate and population-appropriate care, where applicable
- Identification of competency validation method(s) used

- Competency improvement and maintenance activities (staff training, inservices, continuing education, seminars, etc.)

- Most recent education for safety management, hazardous materials and waste, life safety, general safety, and medical equipment usage

- Performance evaluation

TJC also asks surveyors to verify that organizations take a comprehensive approach to collecting competency data and evaluating performance.

Organizations can expect to field surveyor questions regarding their competency assessment process, orientation (including orientation for volunteers), and staff education programs. The box below provides some sample questions surveyors might ask.

The purpose of the competency validation session is to ensure that organizations consistently comply with the standards for staff competency, evaluation, and training. During the competency validation session, surveyors will:

- Review your organization's approach to determining staff qualifications

- Evaluate the orientation, training, and education programs

- Assess the process you use to provide sufficient staff to meet resident/patient needs

- Measure the process you use for evaluating the competency of staff

- Assess the process for incorporating performance evaluations and performance improvement activities.

A variety of issues are addressed during the tracer activity. Surveyors are constantly attuned for examples of situations such as the following:

- Staff discusses the provision of postanesthesia recovery care in more than one location.

- Nurses—in the absence of physical therapists—teach patients how to walk with crutches.

- RNs, LPNs, and respiratory therapists all administering medications.

All such situations lend themselves to the competency discussion because organizations must prove that all disciplines involved in an activity have equal competency to perform the activity in question. It is often these files the surveyors wish to review.

Competency assessment's role in compliance (CMS)

Many organizations choose to provide certain clinical services through outside sources. These sources might or might not provide these services within the organization's facility. Examples of services offered by outside sources may include hemodialysis, lithotripsy, MRI, and cardiac catheterization. Both Centers for Medicare & Medicaid Services (CMS) and TJC have published requirements regarding contract services and the competency of staff. The regulations from the two agencies are remarkably similar. TJC is more descriptive in its requirements regarding the HR aspects of a contract, though CMS certainly alludes to the same expectations. Please note that initial or at-hire competency validation and ongoing competency validation, orientation, and annual performance review are expected for contract staff, just as they are for the organization's direct employees.

Chapter Two

Questions surveyors frequently ask during the competency session:

- What is your vacancy rate for RNs?

- What is the turnover rate?

- What are you doing to recruit and retain RNs?

- What are the three most important things former staff members say would have kept them from leaving?

- Why do staff members tell you they stay?

- What do you do to promote and integrate the various clinical disciplines in understanding their collaborative efforts in quality and safe care delivery?

- How do the leaders of the units/departments determine "ideal" or optimal staffing?

- What benchmarks do you use to analyze the staffing effectiveness indicators you chose?

- Why were those indicators chosen?

- What have you learned from analysis of the staffing effectiveness data?

- With the increase in violence across the nation, what are you doing to prepare the staff, including security staff, for this?

- Walk me through the process of interviewing and making a job offer.

- Describe the process for primary source verification at hire and prior to expiration.

- Tell me about orientation.

- How is competency assessed?

- What about ongoing competency?

Competency assessment tool

Figure 2.1

Name	HR.1.20 Job description	HR.1.20 At hire/prior to expiration primary source licensure/ registration/ certification & verification as required by organization	HR.1.20 Background checks & health screening	HR.2.10 Orientation to organization, unit, and job (only if hired in last three years)	HR.2.10 Orientation to cultural diversity	HR.2.10 Orientation to patient rights—ethical aspects of care	HR.2.10 Ongoing inservice: Safety reporting, team training, population needs	HR.3.10 Competency assessment (qualified individual)	HR.3.20 Performance evaluations Periodically, based on job description—most recent	MS.4.80 Education for recognition of impaired LIPs	NPSG 9.B.4 Fall reduction program education

For each name listed, identify those items at the top of the grid. Make a check mark in the corresponding box, and flag the item in the file. Bring the entire file to the session, including any education files or unit files that may be kept elsewhere.

Chapter three

Six steps to a successful competency program

Six steps to a successful competency program

Introduction

Competency is defined by *Webster's Dictionary* as "the quality of being adequately or well qualified physically and intellectually." Establishing a competency program allows a facility to manage how knowledge, skills, and abilities are incorporated into the performance of an employee.

A well-defined competency program allows managers and employees to work together as a team in order to be successful. When employees clearly understand the expected levels of performance and competency before their hire, they are more likely to become valued members of the team.

Assessing, achieving, and enhancing an employee's competency is an ongoing process. It begins prior to hiring the employees and never ends throughout the tenure of employment. The most effective competency program is one that is integrated into the work environment.

This chapter will assist your facility in the review of your current competency program and provide tips and tools to customize an improved program that will work for you. The pyramid model provides an approach to competency that makes sense and allows for ease of implementation.

There are six levels to achieving competency. Following this approach will provide a foundation of consistency, ease in delivery, and a practical means to improving employee performance and increasing job satisfaction.

Chapter three

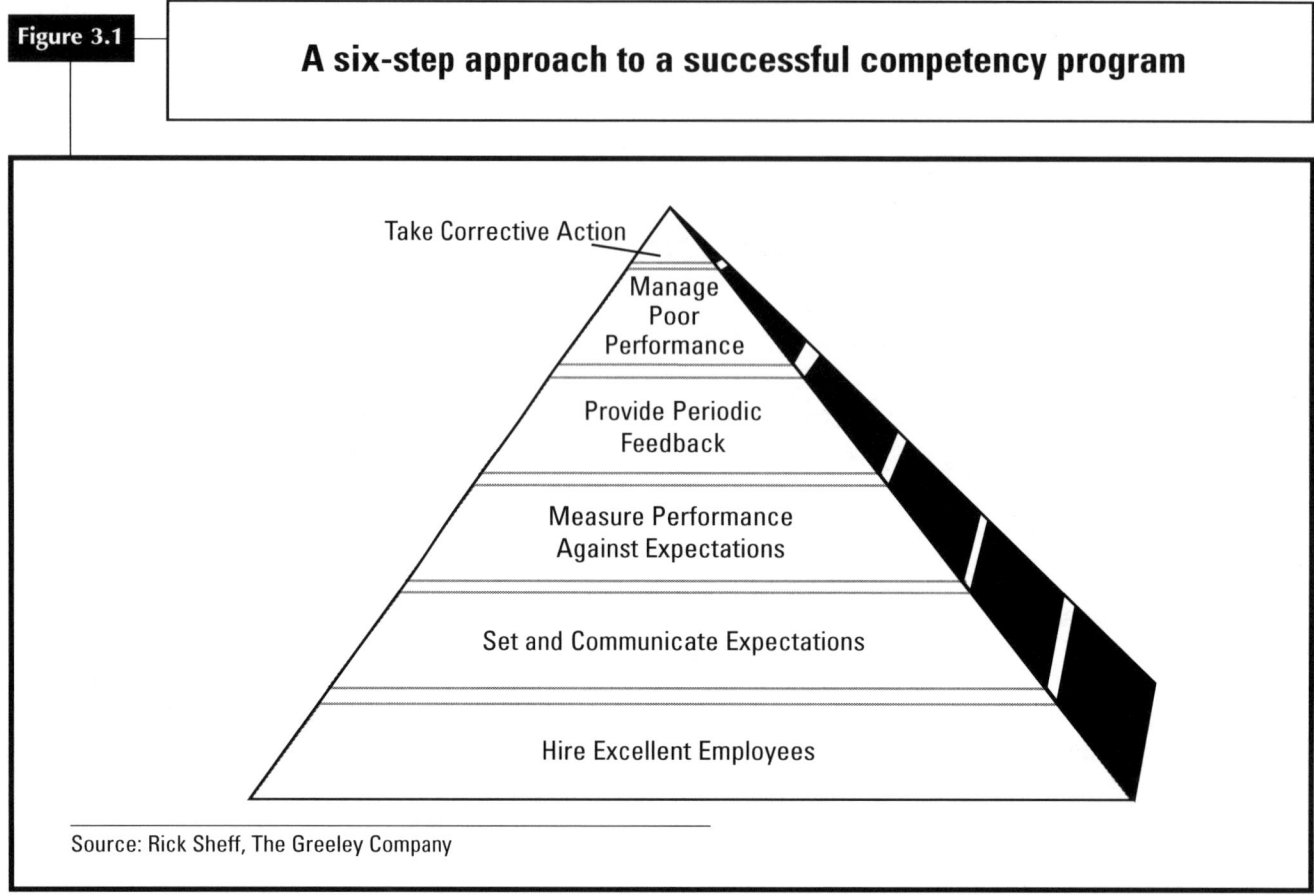

Figure 3.1: A six-step approach to a successful competency program

Source: Rick Sheff, The Greeley Company

Implementing a competency program based on these six steps (see Figure 3.1) in an environment focused on patient safety and professional growth will allow an organization to achieve great performance as well as satisfied employees and customers. These steps apply to all types of healthcare facilities, including acute care, ambulatory care, home health, and long-term care settings.

In an employment market that touts fewer healthcare workers, organizations are challenged to comply with these steps. Staffing shortages and expenses associated with contract employees create an environment of urgency that can lead to hiring individuals who are "less than excellent." A successful competency program is based on a facility's ability to create and maintain the highest possible standards for employees.

Leaders best serve their organization by helping to develop the standards by which each new candidate for employment shall be evaluated. Healthcare facilities are urged to create and maintain the highest possible standards for employees.

Clear and concise advertising for the vacant position can help to reduce time spent on candidates who do not meet the essential requirements. Define the minimum required elements and accept only those applications that meet the requirements.

Job descriptions serve as the foundation of a quality competency program. They provide the starting point for this process. While often considered tedious to develop, a well-researched and well-written job description serves as the basis of control in the hiring process. It should be used to guide the orientation process. The Joint Commission requires hospitals to have a process to ensure that a person's qualifications are consistent with their responsibilities. This requirement is directed at staff members and students, and includes volunteers who work in the same capacity as staff members who provide care, treatment, and service. Leaders of the organization are expected to define the required competency and qualifications of the staff. Job descriptions that are competency-based are the cornerstone in meeting these expectations.

Step 1: Hire excellent employees

Establish competency-based job descriptions
A competency-based job description should include the following requirements:

Job summary
The job summary indicates why the position is in place, the position's relationships to other positions in the department, and the conditions under which the job is performed. The employee should be able to understand his or her relationships to other department members and, if applicable, any employees he or she supervises.

Physical demands
The physical demands should be described in terms of the physical activities (for example, walking, lifting, carrying, pushing, pulling, and bending) that the position entails.

Hierarchy
Define to whom the position reports.

Qualifications
The qualifications component of the job description defines the minimum criteria required to obtain the position. Such criteria include educational requirements; licensure, registration, or certification; and experience.

- The employee must complete an approved training program (dependent on the position). For example, registered nurses (RNs) must graduate from an accredited school of nursing.

- Include required degree level/acceptable number of years of experience. For example, the employee must be an RN, have a bachelor of science degree in nursing (BSN), or be an RN with five years of experience in the area in which he or she is applying.

- Establish required years experience:
    - Clearly define the area of experience. For example, five years' ICU experience.
    - List any special requirements. For example, the employee must be fluent in English and Spanish.

- Provide references from various sources, including professors (if time frame is appropriate), coworkers, and supervisors.

- Request comments on the following:
    - Ability to work well with others
    - Ability to take and give direction
    - Demonstrated commitment to the organization
    - Competency in past position(s)

Competency-based essential elements

- Integrate responsibility and expected practice.

- Incorporate objective, well-defined, and measurable criteria focused on key performance areas.

- Establish basis-of-practice standards that include an age- and/or population-specific component if appropriate.

- Define those tasks that are necessary to the fulfillment of the position. These tasks are used later as the building blocks for competency assessment.

- Review and verify that this list is inclusive before signing off on the job description. Identify the elements the employee must possess prior to being hired, and differentiate them from those that will be developed through training after hiring. Talk with employees who are currently serving in the role to ensure the description and requirements match the actual job.

- Note what population is served.
  - This section should be included in all patient care job descriptions as appropriate. Identification within the job description of the population and ages served offers the new employee the opportunity to assess his or her skills and desire to work with the ages and population defined. Competency as it relates to various age-specific components of assessing, evaluating, treating, and providing care to patients is a Joint Commission expectation.

- Define expectations:
  - Shifts required to work

- Cross training/float requirements

- Professional growth and development expectations and opportunities

Other duties as assigned

- Establish the premise that the job element list is not all-inclusive, and other functions may be added dependent upon certain situations. For example, redistribution of work assignments may occur due to sick call.

- Include expectations such as committee membership, participation in performance improvement projects, role in ensuring a safe environment, required education/classes, and preceptorship, as appropriate.

Review the essential competency-based elements outlined in the job description. Establish an entry-level competency expectation for each of the elements. Communicate with employees the competency expected. For example: Do you expect them to have the basic knowledge of mechanical ventilation, or do you expect them to possess both the basic knowledge and the technical skills required to operate the machine?

Chapter three

During the hiring process, the facility determines whether the applicant has the basic competency to fulfill the position's requirements. For example, a physical therapist who has work experience only in a rehabilitation unit that cared for elderly patients might not have the appropriate background for a pediatric rehabilitation unit. This would warrant further assessment of skills during the interview process.

After the manager makes the decision to hire the applicant, the next step is to validate the information on the application. The Joint Commission requires healthcare organizations to verify the following according to applicable law, regulations, and hospital policy:

- Current licensure, certification, or registration

- Education, experience, and appropriate competency

- Information on criminal background (according to applicable law, regulations, and hospital policy)

- Compliance with healthcare screening requirements that the hospital established

It is important to note that although contract personnel (per diem) and agency personnel are not considered employees, the expectations of competency remain the same. These employment groups should be seamless to the organization regarding the Joint Commission requirements listed above.

Step 1: "Hiring excellent employees" is designed to raise any red flags regarding the potential employee's ability and competency that might require further exploration. Clearly outlining the competency expectation from the beginning is essential to the success of the program. Upon the validation of the application, the entry-level competency assessment is complete.

As children we learned that life was easier when we knew and understood the rules and expectations. This concept carries over into the workplace and is fundamental to hiring excellent employees. When employees know at the time of application what the expectations are for the position, they can make a more educated decision about whether to pursue the process. Expectations are set prior to being hired and are carried throughout the time of employment. Employees need to be provided a clear understanding of what they must do to prepare themselves to be successful. Communication at all levels is the key.

Employees in today's marketplace bring varying knowledge bases and a variety of skills to an organization. However, each facility has its own style and manner of conducting business and setting employee expectations. The ideal forum to begin setting and communicating expectations is through an orientation program.

Establishing an orientation program that is both consistent and effective can be challenging. Managers are often pressed to get people to be willing to address staffing issues. Studies have found that effective orientation programs can improve both retention and satisfaction among employees. If orientation is bypassed, new employees miss the first opportunity to connect with the organization. The organization misses its opportunity to communicate the mission, vision, and expectations to the new employee. Organizational leaders are encouraged to strongly support and require the orientation process. Exceptions should not be granted unless an emergency arises. In this event, critical information must be provided to the employee through another medium. The employee should be scheduled to attend orientation at the next offering.

Step 2: Set and communicate expectations

Establish and maintain an orientation program
Orientation provided to a new employee sets the stage for "setting and communicating expectations." The Joint Commission expects employees to be oriented to their job and work environment prior to providing care, treatment, and services.

Orientation prior to beginning work is an organization's opportunity to let the employees know what is expected of them in the major dimensions of their job performance and competency. These areas include:

- The ability to work well with others including peers, coworkers, visitors, and patients, in all aspects of the job

- Quality of service that is consistent with the organization's mission and vision

- Quality of technical skills

- Appropriate and respectful utilization of resources

- Contribution to the organization and community it serves

Effective orientation programs are usually separated into two very distinct segments—facility orientation and department-specific orientation.

Facility orientation

Often referred to as "general orientation," facility orientation provides a forum where important issues relevant to staff throughout the facility can be presented and discussed with the new staff members. The employees' responsibility to support the organization and to participate actively as a valued member of the staff is established and defined early in their employment.

Facility orientation allows for an overview of organizational policies and procedures that are relevant to all staff members in the organization. The importance of this forum is supported by TJC's requirement that you must orient new employees to the following:

- The facility's mission and goals

- Policies and procedures (including infection control and safety)

- Cultural diversity and sensitivity

- Patient rights and ethical aspects of care

- Infection control

- Safety

- Reporting safety concerns

- Pain management

- National Patient Safety Goals

- Occupational Safety and Health Administration rules and regulations as they apply to staff incidents and injuries

Six steps to a successful competency program

This information is provided to all employees, no matter where they work in the facility, thereby setting both compliance and competency as critical elements to their success.

Facility orientation topics often become the basis for establishing and validating "annual facility-wide competencies."

Typical topics selected for annual competency include the following:

- Mission and vision statement

- National Patient Safety Goals

- Safety of the environment, patients, visitors, and employees

- Infection control

- Corporate integrity

- Patient satisfaction program

- Cultural and religious diversity

- Birth rituals and beliefs

- Family participation

- Dietary practices

- Alternative healthcare approaches

- Death and dying beliefs and practices

- Patient rights

Chapter three

Organizations are challenged to demonstrate the provision of a culture of safety. Staff members are expected to be able to relate what their role and responsibility is as it pertains to safety. The Joint Commission defines this expectation in HR.2.20 by defining four Elements of Performance:

- Risks within the hospital environment

- Action to eliminate, minimize, or report risks

- Procedures to follow in the event of an incident

- Reporting processes for problems, failures, and user errors

Department-specific orientation

Department-specific orientation is used to provide information about the department's activities and responsibilities as well as the employee's responsibilities in the department. The Joint Commission requires facilities to provide specific job duties, responsibilities, and program-specific requirements as a part of orientation. This orientation delves deeper into more specific safety and infection-control practices. Information is provided relevant to the department, age served, specific tasks the employee will be performing, and other areas of responsibility and skills. During the initial days of the department-specific orientation it is important that employee expectations are stressed. New employees can arrive with preconceived notions of what will be expected of them related to job performance and competency. It is the employer's responsibility to define these for the employees.

Department-specific orientation should include the assignment of a mentor or preceptor. The new employee will benefit from knowing he or she has one specific, experienced, and competent individual he or she can rely on to answer questions and guide his or her progress through orientation. It is important that the mentor/preceptor be a peer. Define competency assessment during orientation as well as the time frame in which an employee must meet those expectations.

Entry-level competency, as with all levels of competency assessment, must be conducted by a peer. The Joint Commission qualifies this by stating that "individuals who assess competency are qualified to do so." As such, the director of ancillary services may be a radiology technologist, with laboratory and other services reporting to them. This individual would therefore not be deemed "acceptable" to orient or evaluate the actual bench skill of a medical laboratory technologist, as he or she does not possess the competency.

Successful orientation at the department level requires constant review of content for accuracy and consistency with current practice, process, equipment, and personnel involvement. When a new employee is hired, take the time to review the topics of discussion for the orientation with current staff. A new employee can only be as accurate and competent as the information provided.

Although orientation checklists are not a requirement, documenting the ability of a new employee to fulfill the job expectations is mandatory. Joint Commission 2008 standard HR.2.10 includes Elements of Performance that address the required components of the initial hospital orientation program. These elements include topics such as:

- Mission and goals of the organization

- Hospital policies and procedures
    - Safety
    - Infection control
    - Unit- and/or program-specific

- Cultural diversity and sensitivity

- Patient rights and ethics and the processes used to address these issues

Many organizations have found an outline or guide of topics to cover is useful (See figure 3.2).

Throughout the orientation period, and as part of the ongoing competency program, the incorporation of population-specific components is required (See Figure 3.3).

Figure 3.2 — **Example of portion of department-specific guidelines**

	DEPARTMENT ORIENTATION	
Tour	• Nursing station • Utility room(s) • Nourishment center • Waiting area • Equipment storage	• Supplies—medical and office • Medication room(s) • Fire extinguisher(s) • Medical gas valve
Routine	• Phone, fax, copier, pager, and computer programs • Access codes to various areas • Location of physician and employee phone/pager list, call roster, etc. • Material safety data sheets (computer or notebook)	• Messenger/tube system • Crash cart(s)—frequency of checks and operation of equipment • Housekeeping, bed cleaning, etc.
Documentation	• Chart order • Electronic record • Banned abbreviations • All patient care forms and guidelines for completion • Request forms—equipment repair, dietary, laboratory, radiology, etc.	• Consents • Data collection tools • Incident reports, adverse drug reaction reports • Medication record • Medication scanning
Process	• Patient identifiers • Handoff process • Telephone orders • Patient transport • Code, including defibrillation • Fall-reduction program • Rapid response team • Core measure compliance • Critical value results and tests • Medication reconciliation • Protocol implementation • Universal Protocol	• Notification of infection control • Moderate sedation—bedside procedures requiring "time-out" and documentation requirements • IV, phlebotomy • Point-of-care testing • Restraints • Care guides, preprinted orders
Population served	• Age-specific components • Interpreter services • Assessment • Psychosocial factors	• Safety • Education • Environment

Figure 3.3 — Sampling of population-specific components

Geriatric Populations	
Assessment	Physical assessments include vital signs, weight, skin assessment, signs of neglect or abuse, nutritional needs.
Psychosocial	Ensure availability of communication devices (e.g., hearing aids, glasses). Communication with patient reflects knowledge that feelings of worth, pride, and usefulness need to be maintained. Reduce fear of being left alone. Inclusion of family is important to ensure continuity of care.
Safety	Take precautions to prevent falls Watch for signs of "sundowning" and take precautions as appropriate
Medication Management	Review medication dosages to ensure appropriate doses due to degenerative changes in body functions.
Physically Challenged	
Assessment	Physical assessments as per routine with additional attention related to skin issues from prosthesis, crutches, etc.
Psychosocial	Provide education and support in an age-appropriate manner. (Physically challenged does not equal mentally challenged.) Reassure patient to reduce likelihood of being self-conscious and embarrassed.
Safety	Ensure the environment is free from obstacles to reduce risk of falls Ensure proper equipment is readily available to allow for safe independence.

Populations to be addressed could include such groups as:

- Geriatric
- Pediatric
- Special needs such as hearing or sight impaired
- Physically challenged
- Developmentally or emotionally challenged

Other population-/age-specific topics to include in the competency program should include as appropriate:

- Proper equipment selection based on size and age
- Restraints
- Knowledge of acceptable medication dosages based on age and weight
- Psychosocial considerations based on age and environmental factors
- Safety, including the fall-risk assessment and reduction strategies defined by the organization
- Learning styles and opportunities

These population-specific components should be assessed at entry level and ongoing as an element of core competencies, as appropriate.

Assessing entry-level competency can help to streamline and individualize the orientation and training for the new employee. Self-assessment is often used as a tool to begin this process. While this tool may have some value, it is often difficult to validate how the new employee interprets his or her skill level. Successful organizations have found it to be much more valuable to test entry competency based on the organization's established expectations and competency validation assessments. Be cautious when utilizing a self-assessment tool. Failure to ensure competency assessment follow-up when an employee has indicated on a self-assessment the need for "further instruction or review" can be a failure of a competency process.

Validating competency during the orientation process can be challenging. Begin with the end in mind: The manner in which competency is evaluated after orientation should mirror the manner in which competency will be assessed throughout the employee's tenure. Establish a monitoring system that will assist in letting both the manager and the new employee know where opportunities to improve exist.

> **Step 2:** "Set and communicate expectations" is designed to ensure new employees are welcomed into the organization with a quality, comprehensive, and pertinent orientation. Adequately oriented employees are provided the tools necessary to be successful. When expectations are set and communicated at the beginning of employment, the outcome will be safe and competent care/service.

The art of measuring employee performance against expectations becomes less overwhelming when excellent employees have been hired and adequately oriented.

Measuring performance against expectations requires a process of establishing and maintaining performance expectations. Competency is defined by such adjectives as capability, skill, proficiency, experience, and expertise. It is the ability of an employee to integrate his or her knowledge, skill, experience, and attitude when performing an assessment/procedure/documentation.

Create a monitoring system that can bring to employees' attention aspects of their performance that represent variations from expectations. This will help to remove the subjective information that so often distorts evaluations of performance.

Step 3: Measure performance against expectations

Define and create a monitoring system

Before performance expectations can be assessed, it is important to clarify what specific Elements of Performance will be measured and where the data will be obtained. As has been a theme throughout this chapter, expectation aids in the consistency and communication of measurement.

Data used to measure performance can be found in numerous sources.

Examples of data sources are:

- Incident reports.

- Care-guide reports that reflect deviation from clinical pathways. Clinical pathways are multidisciplinary care plans that have been developed based on best clinical practices for specified groups of patients with a particular diagnosis. Clinical pathways facilitate the coordination and delivery of high-quality care.

- Patient satisfaction surveys.

- Medication error reports.

- Chart audit tools.

- Supervisor observation.

Competency-based performance assessment challenges organizations to use both internal and external benchmarks and resist the urge to review performance based on an employee's ability to accurately complete a document. Competency is assessed from the content of the document rather than the document itself. For example, proper completion of a discharge form, while important, does not assess competency to adequately prepare a patient for discharge. Properly identifying barriers to discharge and enlisting appropriate and authorized resources to facilitate removal of the barriers demonstrates an employee's competency in knowledge, planning, and appropriate utilization of resources. To assess competency at this level, an organization must have implemented care guides or pathways that trigger variance reports when not followed properly.

Thorough review of medication errors, including practitioner-specific information, is also vital. It is essential for an organization's processes that it uses such data collected—when practitioner-specific—as a means to identify opportunities for additional training and mentorship. Root-cause analysis of why errors occur, more often than not, reveals the process is "at fault" or contributory to the practitioner error.

Competency assessment of every skill, task, knowledge base, or process that an employee may need is simply not possible. Core competencies should be established to determine an employee's performance against measures that are based on skills and tasks that fall into one or more of the following categories:

- High-volume

- High-risk

- Problem-prone

Each department manager evaluates the activities in his or her service area and selects the skills, tasks, and processes that fall into the above three categories. Measuring performance of core competencies based on actual performance is essential to assessing the competency of employees. The selection of core competencies should be based on the results of aggregated and trended data from a variety of sources, including:

- Performance improvement activities

- Infection-control reports

- Safety reports

- Risk-management reports

- Equipment user-error reports

- New or expanding technology

- Policy and procedures changes

- Strategic plan initiatives

The annual competency assessment process is not comprehensive like the competency validation that occurs during orientation. Once the employee has demonstrated that he or she has knowledge and the ability necessary to perform the position's assigned responsibilities, tasks, and skills, competency is established.

Although managers consider basic competencies for annual competency verification, it is critical for managers to select the elements that are important enough to include in the annual competency program. Typically, three to five competencies will be selected for review each year.

Chapter three

Managers use a variety of resources to help them choose annual competencies. These may include:

- Department functions

- Performance improvement activities

- Infection-control reports

- New technology

- Any activity that is important to the success of the department

Another creative strategy is to ask the employees, "What patient or disease process are you the most uncomfortable caring for?" Once answers are identified, assist the employees in further defining what elements they are most uncomfortable with. It may be the equipment you're using in caring for the patient, the disease process itself, or the emotional or psychological components involved. Whatever the reason, design a competency program that will address those issues and provide a meaningful outcome that is employee-driven.

A word of caution: Do not confuse "comfort" with "competency." An employee may be fully competent to care for a patient and not feel comfortable. Be aware of the distinct difference and ensure the process addresses the competency, which will then, by design, increase the comfort level.

The review process of defining the selection of annual competencies can be simplified into four categories (See Figure 3.4)

- New duties

- Problem-prone

- Low-volume/high-risk

- Monitoring component

Six steps to a successful competency program

| Figure 3.4 | **Review process categories** |

The following categories are annual competencies to be reviewed:

- **New duties**—Example: A home-health program has introduced a new wound-vacuum system and increased IV therapy treatments by 50% in the age groups of children and the elderly in the last six months. The chosen competency is the education of the patient and family/caregiver, and where to document both the patient data and education in the computerized medical record.

- **Problem-prone**—Example: Following the communitywide disaster drill, it was noted that staff members were unaware of how to contact the command center, complete the appropriate paperwork, and obtain adequate supplies. Re-education of the disaster preparedness program is selected as the competency.

- **Low-volume and high-risk**—Example: Only two children entered the emergency department in respiratory distress in the last six months. The chosen competency for respiratory therapists is the response to pediatric respiratory emergencies. Procedures requiring the use of moderate sedation occurred only three times in the past year, requiring this to become a competency for nursing.

- **Activities/responsibilities mandated for ongoing competency**—Activities identified as part of the department monitoring systems/performance improvement/infection control and/or mandated for ongoing competency. Example: The performance improvement monitoring system identified errors in the waived testing proficiency findings. Restraint data revealed an increased use of restraints without proper documentation. These topics were selected as competencies to address the regulatory performance requirements.

Timely performance reviews

Leaders, managers, or directors must meet with employees to review their performance within a defined period. The Joint Commission requires that this review take place at least once within the three-year accreditation cycle. Once the review time frame has been established, all managers, leaders, and directors must commit to conducting timely performance reviews for all employees who report to them.

Chapter three

> **Step 3:** "Measure performance against expectations" is designed to ensure a systematic approach to identifying and measuring key performance elements that ensure the provision of care or service by competent individuals.

When employees do excellent work, provide quality care, and exhibit superior customer service, they deserve feedback. The converse is also true. When expectations are not met and patient satisfaction is compromised, this must also be communicated. Establishing a system that provides routine feedback to employees regarding their performance as measured against expectations is essential to a competency program.

Most healthcare organizations, in response to previously established Joint Commission standards, had required an annual performance appraisal. This standard was changed in 2004 to at least once in a three-year period of time. Careful review of the rationale stated for this change in 2004 reveals the phrase "ongoing process." Performance feedback should be offered in an ongoing manner that includes both what the employee is performing at or above expectations in and also those performance elements that are falling short of the required standard, allowing employees to identify areas of learning and growth potential. Feedback that is data-based allows employees to further evaluate their performance against both expectations and peers.

Step 4: Provide periodic feedback

Establish a means of conducting ongoing performance review
A performance review process that is both ongoing and interactive can be rewarding as well as exciting, and will ultimately be the key to maintaining competent employees. Employee performance data that are communicated using graphic tools can have more impact. Remember in Step 2 that clear expectations were communicated. In this step, performance is expected to be reviewed and communicated, ultimately leading to increased competency.

Data that are displayed graphically are not necessarily more easily understood. Imagine if information regarding medication errors were to be presented as in Figure 3.5.

Does this graph provide an employee with the ability to assess his or her competency related to medication management? Can the manager expect a change in performance that will result in the reduction of errors based on this display of data? What if the data looked like the graph represented in Figure 3.6?

Six steps to a successful competency program

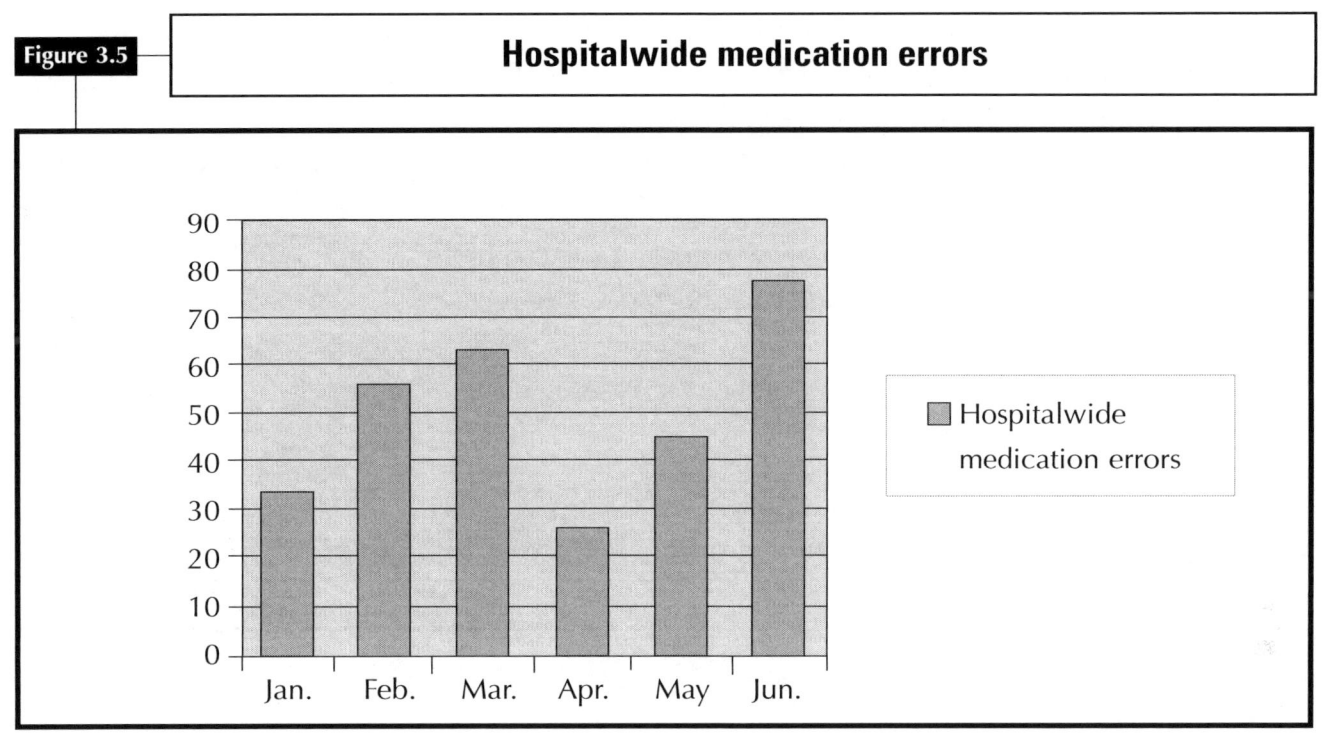

Figure 3.5 — Hospitalwide medication errors

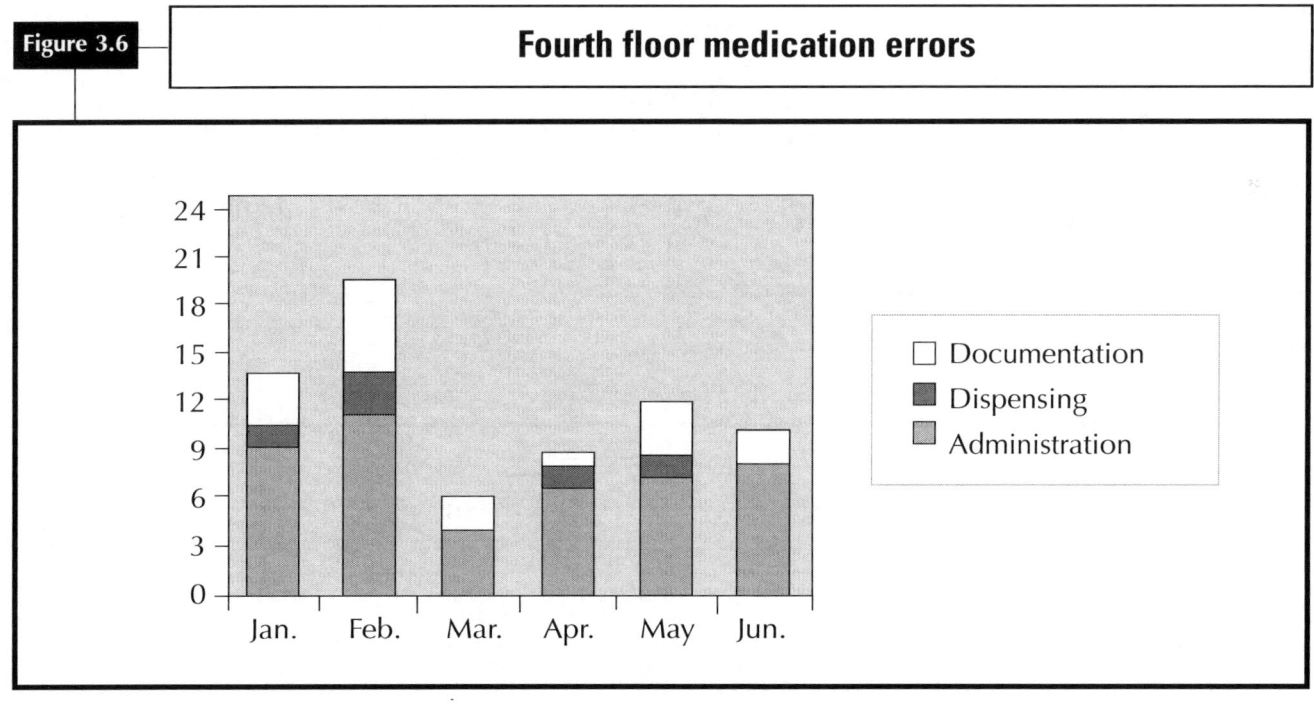

Figure 3.6 — Fourth floor medication errors

The information provided in this graph begins to clearly communicate the opportunities for improvement, as specific to one area of the organization. Feedback provided in this manner allows the team the opportunity to begin to prioritize areas of improvement. The area where performance is meeting expectations is displayed to provide positive feedback and encouragement.

The initial collection of the performance data can be accomplished using well-defined data elements. Organizations need to decide how much data detail they will collect. Collecting more initial information reduces the need to re-review charts or other data sources. Once an improvement focus is identified, further drill-down of the data can begin. For example, Figure 3.7 represents the data in an even further-defined manner.

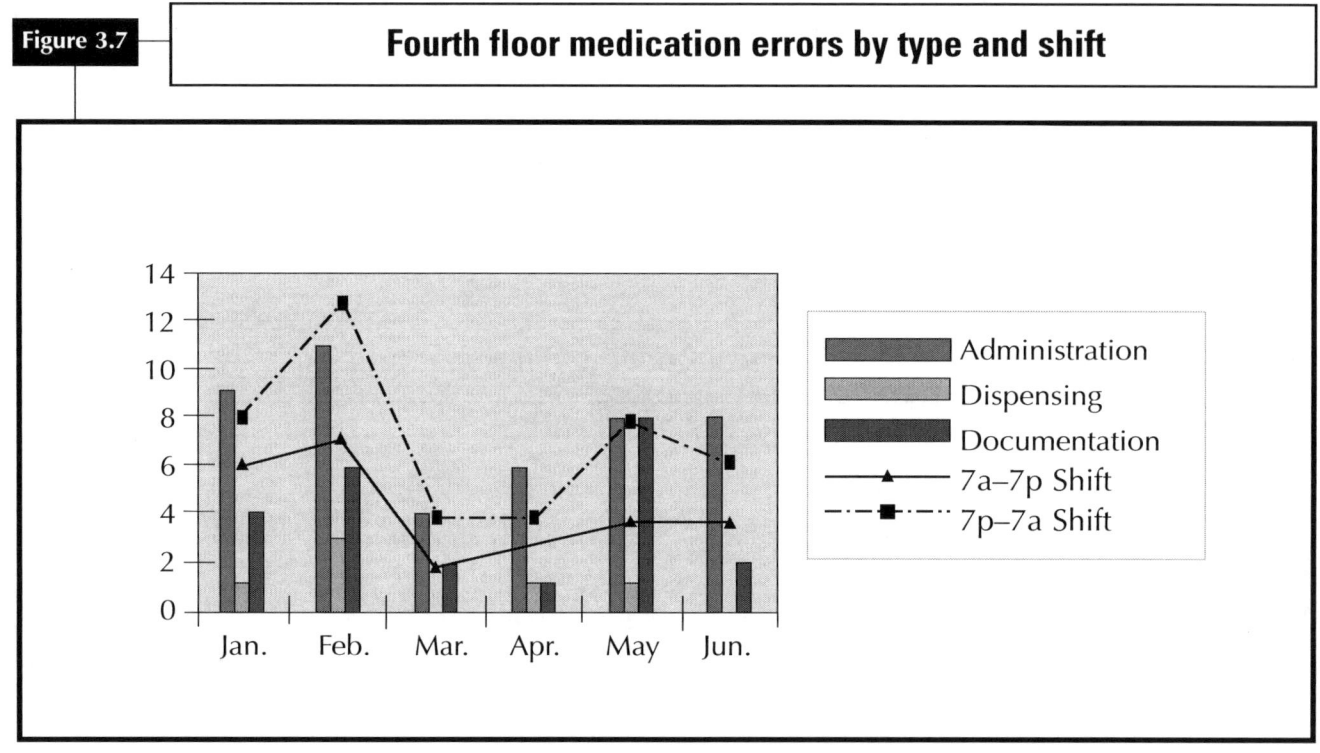

Figure 3.7 **Fourth floor medication errors by type and shift**

Employees now can review these data and clearly identify the greatest impact on improvement.

This type of ongoing performance feedback enhances a competency program by providing feedback that measures performance against expectations. Feedback that is timely allows employees to review the issues and make corrective changes before their overall performance is compromised. Performance feedback is focused on process, not the person, which increases the likelihood of improvement as employees can relate the impact of performance to patient outcomes without feeling personally attacked.

Managers are encouraged to assess what motivates their employees to improve. Utilization of creative improvement strategies such as unit challenges or challenges between shifts allows a competency program to provide feedback in an environment that encourages improvement and stimulates growth, thereby validating or improving competency.

> **Step 4:** "Providing periodic feedback," when implemented in a consistent manner, praises individuals or groups for quality performance and provides a positive atmosphere when opportunities for improvement are identified. Employeeswho work in this setting help each other to be the best healthcare providers possible.

Step 5: Manage poor performance

Establish future goals and improvement targets

Manage poor performance in order to embrace improvement opportunities. Help employees be the best they can be rather than trying to catch them in the wrong. Managing performance is the equivalent of managing results. An employee not meeting expectations should have an opportunity to improve his or her performance. Try the following process:

- Establish the goal

- Determine how problems will be verified
    - Refer to data

- Understand what it will take to meet the expectations
    - Define the variables

- Have a toolkit ready to resolve the problems

- Know how to measure progress toward the goal
    - Measure effectiveness (doing the right thing)
    - Measure efficiency (doing things right)

- Clearly set the "reward" of goal achievement

Chapter three

1. Establish the goal
It is important to remember that the goal of managing poor performance is ultimately to improve the performance. Setting performance targets, reviewing the measures necessary to meet the target, and accurately and systematically measuring the outcomes are keys to success.

2. Determine how problems will be verified
Address the "behavior" rather than the person when assisting employees to develop collaborative and team approaches to working together. Referring to the data, as opposed to reinforcing the errors, allows employees to stay focused on achieving the goal and improving their competency. Manage the poor performance by managing for results.

3. Understand what it will take to meet the expectations
Before competency can be improved, it is important to understand what variables/barriers exist. Explore the following:

- Knowledge base

- Skill set

- Environmental factors

- Personal issues

4. Have a toolkit ready to resolve the problems
Be innovative and persistent when managing poor performance. Ask the employee to complete a self-assessment on motivation (See Figure 3.8). What drives the employee to succeed? Structure the improvement of the competency around the employee's motivation and energy.

Figure 3.8 — **Sample questions for self-assessment of motivation**

1. What do you do best?
2. What are your weaknesses? What steps have you taken to improve your knowledge and/or skill?
3. What special talents do you have?
4. What would you like to improve or learn more about?
5. What do you enjoy doing? (e.g., writing, researching, problem solving, helping others, etc.)
6. What would you prefer not to do? Is this because of comfort or competence?
7. What are some of the things that energize you and give you satisfaction?
8. What task- or job-related issues are important to you? (e.g., autonomy, problem solving, challenge, variety, structure, money, job security, flexibility, promotion, personal development)
9. What people-related things are important to you? (e.g., helping and supporting others, working alone, honesty, teamwork, open communication)
10. What ideas do you have regarding "service recovery"?
11. What environment-related things are important to you? (e.g., industry, workplace culture, physical environment)
12. How do you interact with people?
13. What is your approach to tasks?
14. What kinds of information do you naturally notice? Factors to consider include:
    - Decisiveness
    - Temperament
    - Levels of assertiveness or agreeableness, tact
    - Need for social interaction
    - Social confidence
    - Rule awareness
    - Impulsiveness
    - Persuasiveness
    - Intuition
    - Levels of patience or tolerance
    - Open-mindedness
    - Self-discipline
    - Levels of perfectionism
    - Anxiety

5. Know how to measure progress toward the goal

Establish a measurement system that will clearly demonstrate how achieving the goal will be assessed. Effectiveness and efficiency are keys to success. Benchmarking progress toward a goal is important so the employee can visualize his or her success or need for additional improvement. "Do the right thing and do things right" should be the mantra for improvement.

6. Clearly set the "reward" for goal achievement

Create an additional reward other than retained employment. Successfully managing poor performance can lead to improved processes, staffing adjustments, barrier removal, and increased job satisfaction. Improving a process during performance management can be beneficial to all members of the team.

> Step 5: "Managing poor performance" should be a very small segment of a competency program. Periodic performance feedback provides both managers and employees the "heads up" needed to prevent poor performance from reaching a level of required individual action. Incorporating the lessons learned when managing poor performance into the competency plan will further assist in decreasing the need to address this segment of the pyramid.

Step 6: Take corrective action

When care is compromised, corrective action is needed

Consistently follow the previous steps of a successful competency program to ensure that Step 6 will be a very small component of your program. The step is necessary when performance fails to improve/meet expectations. When patient care is jeopardized, organizational leaders are required to take corrective action. Except in extreme cases or when laws are broken, corrective action should be the last step in a well-designed program.

Taking corrective action may involve professional leadership from the human resources department. Ensure all appropriate policies and procedures are followed and that the employee's rights are protected.

Conclusion

A competency program that is based on the six-step approach will require commitment from leadership throughout an organization. Extra resources may at times be necessary but worthwhile.

The Joint Commission continues to test the effectiveness of the competency program through the tracer methodology. Interviews with staff and subsequent reviews of personnel files allow surveyors to make a determination of compliance with the requirements of the Elements of Performance. Employees who can clearly articulate the orientation and competency assessment processes demonstrate how the organization is meeting the requirements. Personnel files that reflect documentation supporting the concepts of the six-step approach reinforce the culture of the organization and can lead to a successful survey.

"It is the nature of man to rise to greatness **if greatness is expected** of him."
—John Steinbeck (1902–1968)

Chapter four

What is the competency validation cycle?

What is the competency validation cycle?

Competency validation is the process of ensuring that each employee possesses the skill set identified in the job description and adequately performs the tasks or activities for his or her position according to an established standard. Organizations validate competency not only to comply with regulatory requirements, including those of Centers for Medicare & Medicaid Services (CMS) and The Joint Commission (TJC), but also to ensure that employees perform the duties appropriate to their job descriptions.

The competency validation cycle has three phases or three situations with different intents in which the organization verifies competency. These are as follows:

- At hire (initial)
- End of the orientation period
- Ongoing basis

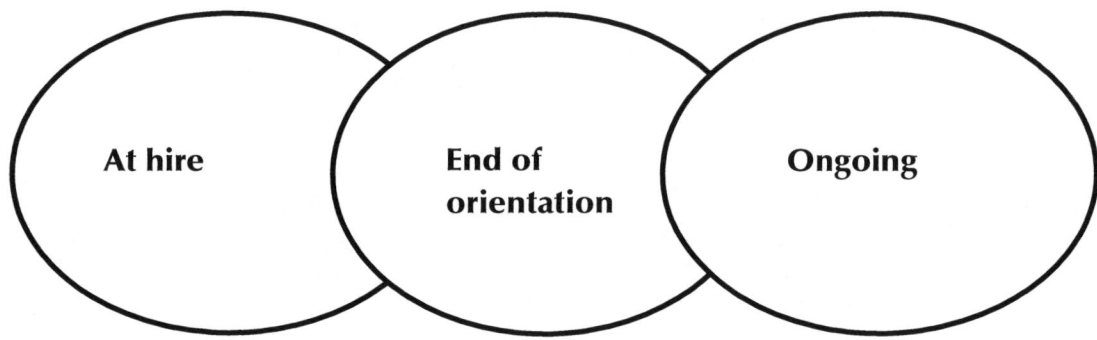

CHAPTER FOUR

At-hire competency validation

What is at-hire competency validation?

At-hire or initial competency validation begins when an individual applies for a position at the organization. Before hiring an applicant, an organization must verify that the applicant meets all the qualifications specified in the job description, including any required education, license, registration, certification, experience, special skills, knowledge, and abilities, and that the individual has a satisfactory criminal background check and satisfactory references from previous employers, if applicable. In many organizations, this is a shared responsibility between the staff in the human resources department and the leader of the unit/department interested in filling a position. In other organizations, this function may be carried out entirely by the human resources staff. Either option is acceptable, but the responsibility should be defined in organizational policy.

For whom must organizations perform at-hire competency validation?

Organizations must validate at-hire competency for all prospective employees, students, and volunteers serving in the same capacity as paid staff. Initial competency validation for students is completed by the educational program at which the student is matriculating. The organization should ensure that the educational institution performed primary-source verification of the clinical faculty accompanying students present in the organization. At-hire competency validation must be completed for all staff members, including both direct employees and contract employees, and for both clinical and nonclinical staff members.

Individuals are direct employees if the organization hires and pays them. In many organizations, direct employees compose the entire work force. Direct employees include those who work in nursing, environmental services, the business office, the pharmacy, and medical records.

On occasion, some organizations decide to outsource a clinical department or service. In this case, another entity provides the care or service to the organization's patients through a contractual arrangement. A few examples of such contracted services and departments might include hemodialysis, lithotripsy, and nuclear medicine. In other situations, the organization may provide the service itself but have difficulty hiring a sufficient number of individuals to fill the positions needed to staff the service or department. In this case, the organization may contract with an employment agency to provide the needed staffing for the department or service. These arrangements may be temporary in nature or may extend over a long period of time. All or part of the staff providing the care, treatment, or service may be actual employees of the agency rather than of the organization. As such, they are paid by the agency itself rather than by the organization "purchasing" their services from the agency. Organizations must validate the qualifications of employees of outside agencies—such employees are often referred to as contract employees—following the same process as that used for the direct employees, although responsibilities may be shared between the agency and the organization.

Please note that organizations must also validate competency for physicians and for allied health professionals (i.e., physician assistants, nurse practitioners, etc.), but they do so through an entirely separate process—the credentialing and privileging process—which is outside the scope of this book.

Verifying qualifications

An organization usually verifies education by reviewing what the applicant stated on his or her application, but some organizations prefer to view diplomas or to verify completion of educational programs with the schools the applicant has listed.

A critical component of initial competency verification is primary source verification, which is discussed in detail in Chapter 1.

Organizations should verify qualifications, including licensure, registration, or certification for all staff members, not only for those who provide direct patient care. It is important to keep in mind that there are some non-clinical positions that require a license, registration, or certification to carry out the essential functions of the job. For example, a driver in the transportation department must possess a current, valid driver's license.

At-hire competency validation is complete when the organization has verified all qualifications specified for the job. If this is a shared process between HR staff and the unit/department leader, HR staff share their findings with the appropriate department manager so that this information can be used at the time the hiring decision is made. If the applicant does not meet the required qualifications, the organization should not hire the applicant unless there is a documented attribute that the candidate will bring to the organization that outweighs the lack of one or more required qualifications. For example, an individual might lack experience but possess an advanced educational degree in a field the organization deems critical. Such an attribute should be so compelling as to negate the importance of his or her lack of any qualifications specified for the position.

Integrating at-hire competency validation into the hiring process

Organizations usually pick one of two ways to integrate at-hire verification into the hiring process. Some organizations prefer to verify all necessary information before the applicant interviews with his or her prospective unit/department leader. Other organizations prefer to verify some of the qualifications, interview the applicant, and then complete the validation process.

Whichever method an organization chooses, it should define the process in its HR policy. The HR policy should also define the process the organization uses to:

- Orient new employees
- Validate competency after orientation
- Conduct periodic performance reviews
- Validate ongoing competency

Competency validation during the orientation period

Organizations must provide orientation to all new staff members, students, and volunteers serving in the same capacity as staff members. It is during orientation that the organization introduces individuals to policies, procedures, and processes, as well as to tasks they must perform and equipment they will be expected to use with skill.

Some of the policies, procedures, and processes addressed during orientation are determined by the requirements of regulatory agencies such as the Occupational Safety and Health Administration (OSHA), TJC, and the Centers for Disease Control and Prevention (CDC). Other items covered in orientation reflect organization-specific decisions about the topics with which the organization thinks all employees/volunteers should be familiar.

It is also during orientation that the unit/department leader has an opportunity to determine whether the employee—including those providing care, treatment, or service under a contractual arrangement or as a volunteer—can carry out the essential responsibilities of the job and is competent to perform the job.

Competency must also include determining whether the employee can provide care in an age-appropriate or population-appropriate manner if such modifications must be made in assessment/evaluation/treatment of patients—sometimes referred to as direct-care delivery or clinical-care delivery. Examples of staff members who provide clinical care, treatment, or service for which there is an age-related aspect to the activity include RN/LPN, physical therapists, clinical dietitians, pharmacists, etc. However, for many activities carried out by clinical staff members no expectation exists that the activities be performed in a different way if the patient receiving the care, treatment, or service is of a certain age or population group. Likewise, responsibilities of nonclinical staff members have no age-related aspect to them at all, as these staff members are not providing care, treatment, or service to patients.

The job description should identify the age groups/population groups to which the employee will be expected to provide care. The organization should determine whether any of the responsibilities required of the individual have an age-related aspect to them. If so, competency validation must include verification that this activity is modified as indicated in a policy, procedure, algorithm, standard of care or practice, guideline, or some other resource. These resources for how the activity is to be carried out can be thought of as the "rule" and serve as the foundation for competency validation.

See Chapter 5 for descriptions of the various methods organizations can use to validate competency.

Ongoing competency validation

What is ongoing competency validation?

Ongoing competency validation is the continued demonstration by all employees, students, and volunteers serving in the same capacity as staff of their ability to perform the essential responsibilities of the job for which they were hired. They typically fall into one or more of the following categories:

- Essential job functions that are performed with high frequency

- Essential but rarely performed job functions

- Job functions that have proven problematic for individuals or groups of staff members

- Job functions that one or more regulatory agencies require the organization to review on an annual basis and in which staff members are required to demonstrate ongoing competency in performing, regardless of the frequency with which they are performed, or the problem-free aspect of the activity

- Recently introduced or modified job functions

Once staff members complete orientation, they begin to function without direct supervision as they carry out the functions of their job. Employees demonstrate ongoing competency by performing their essential or primary responsibilities on a frequent basis as a regular part of doing their jobs. For these frequently occurring activities that are performed without change, data already being collected by many organizations for some other purpose can be used to assess ongoing competency.

Competency can be assessed through reviewing data gathered from regular job performance. For example, the medication-error monitoring performed by all hospitals follows the idea that as long as the process being assessed through data collection, aggregation, and analysis is in statistical control, the individuals performing those activities are demonstrating their competency.

Such data sources include risk management reports (patient falls, employee back injuries, sharps exposures), medication-error reports, sentinel-event and proactive risk assessments (failure modes and effects analysis), unit/department monitoring and evaluation activities as a part of organizational performance improvement (PI), patient-satisfaction surveys, complaint logs, critiques following all drills and mock events (such as fire drills, mock codes, etc.), and critiques following actual events, (such as loss of utilities following a hurricane, tornado, or flood). Other data may also be available. Managers do not necessarily need to create or request new or additional reports to verify continued competency in unchanged core responsibilities or to identify areas requiring improvement; they simply need to examine the information already available to them through quality monitoring and evaluation efforts.

On occasion, a review of aggregate data will indicate that a process is out of statistical control. In this situation, the organizational leaders should identify where the opportunity for improvement lies. If it is determined the opportunity lies with staff performance rather than with the design of the process, this opportunity for improvement should be pursued. It usually involves reeducating applicable staff about the steps of the process identified as a problem, then validating competency.

Some activities, while critical to a job, may occur infrequently. We call these low-volume activities. Because they occur infrequently, existing data cannot be used to demonstrate ongoing competency. The activity may have been performed by no one, or, at best, by a limited number of staff members during a defined period of time, usually a year. Statistical sampling theory suggests that another method of ensuring ongoing competency must be used when volume of any activity is insufficient for a review of existing data to be a valid method for ongoing competency validation. The decision as to what sufficient volume is should be made by unit/department leaders.

Certain regulatory agencies have requirements regarding the frequency with which staff must receive education and validate their competency to perform activities essential to their job. These agencies specify annual education and validation of a competency. These requirements have applicability for staff regardless of the frequency with which they are performed and regardless of past demonstrations of competency.

During any given year, many organizations introduce new technologies and improvements in existing technology, new medications and treatments, and new ways to perform procedures more efficiently and effectively. Consequently, jobs often change during the course of a year. Whether the change is a new process, a new piece of equipment, a new task, or a new way to perform an old task, any affected employee must be educated about the change as it occurs. Following the employee's orientation to the change, the organization must validate the employee's competency in carrying out the new aspect of his or her job. Because such a validation occurs in direct response to a change, and at the time of such a change, it is referred to as ongoing competency validation. Some of these changes affecting clinical staff have an age-related or population-related aspect to them, so competency validation must include verification that the individual can competently modify the process when indicated by patient age or population.

Identifying ongoing competencies

Unit/department leaders must identify the responsibilities for which staff, students, and volunteers must demonstrate ongoing competency. It requires the leader to develop a list of responsibilities for which the employee must demonstrate ongoing competency. To do this, the leader should set aside some time for planning prior to the start of "the year," as defined by the organization. Some use the calendar year; others the fiscal year. In advance of the "new year," ongoing competencies to evaluate must be identified. The identified set of competencies reflects the plans of the leader and allows for unplanned activities to occur during the year. The leader needs to have access to aggregate data reports, strategic plans for the organization/his or her department, organizational and departmental goals, and the approved budget for the coming year, as he or she starts the planning process. These should all be considered when identifying ongoing competencies.

The planning process begins with a review of the job description. The primary responsibilities of the job and the populations and age group(s) for whom care, treatment, or service is provided are identified. If any of these are anticipated to change in the coming year, changes are made to the job description at this time.

Available aggregate data reports should be reviewed by the leader in order to verify ongoing competency of staff, students, and volunteers for those primary responsibilities that are high-volume in nature and for which a data source exists. Aggregate data is the term TJC uses for data an organization compiles and reviews over a long period of time. Sources of aggregate data include risk management reports, customer satisfaction reports, medication error reports, and infection control reports (see Chapter 6 for further discussion of aggregate data). Although these reports were reviewed during the year in order to identify any unplanned opportunities for staff education and demonstration of competency as problems were identified, the data for the past year are reviewed in order to identify competencies that may need to be assessed for the coming year. We call these problem-prone activities.

The leader reviews the primary responsibilities in order to identify any that are low in volume. Because the activity occurs infrequently, aggregate data cannot be used either as the measure of ongoing competency or to identify a lack of ongoing competency, since sufficient volume of the activity is not present. So at least an annual review of the expectations of how the process is to be carried out is needed, followed by an assessment of competency of staff members carrying out the activity as a part of their job. Such validation helps ensure that employees maintain competency in areas in which they have less opportunity to use those skills.

The primary responsibilities are then reviewed to determine which duties are mandated by an external regulatory agency or by the organization as a validation requirement each year, regardless of the frequency with which they are performed and regardless of past demonstrations of competency.

Determine the changes expected in the coming year and how these changes will affect employee job functions in a particular unit/department in order to validate job responsibilities in the coming year. This may represent anticipated changes in technology, equipment, services, programs, processes, policies, procedures, and patient populations to which staff will be expected to provide care or services. Education will need to be planned for staff affected by the planned changes, followed by more competency validation.

Some of the responsibilities on the ongoing competency list will have an age-related aspect to how they are to be performed. Leaders should identify these responsibilities just as they do when validating competency at the end of orientation. Organizations also use the same methodologies for validating ongoing competency as they use for validating competency at the end of the orientation period. Please see Chapter 5 for descriptions of the various validation methodologies.

Many leaders find it helpful to develop a plan for when staff will be educated or reeducated about the identified responsibilities on the list, and their competency validated. In keeping with the concept of ongoing competency, this planning should occur at various times during the coming year. A logical place to start is with a review of existing educational and competency validation dates already developed by the organization's education department. These activities are designed to allow staff members to receive education and validate competency for those activities that are mandated on an annual basis and may also be planned in response to identified problems that affect a significant number of staff members. Assigning various times for staff members to attend is then a simple matter. The date an existing process is scheduled to change or a new process is scheduled to begin should already be identified in the organization's strategic plan or department/unit goals. Staff education and competency validation should be planned to precede implementation of the change or new process/equipment being introduced. A time must be allocated to reeducate staff about expectations for any low-volume responsibilities on the list. The leader of the unit/department presents the educational material and validates staff competency or negotiates with someone else to do this. Scheduling all these activities before the year begins allows the leader to respond to the need to educate staff members and validate competency for those unplanned events that may occur within the year.

When do managers assess ongoing competencies?

The formal review of competency usually occurs at the same time as the employee's performance review. While people often consider the two processes to be one and the same, they are not the same. Ongoing competency validation reflects the employee's continued ability to perform his or her job in a competent fashion, even as the job changes. Competency is always about the job and is specific to the activities/responsibilities of the job, whatever that job may be. Performance expectations are not job-specific. They are expectations of all staff, regardless of the job. The annual performance review reflects the employee's ability to meet the contractual or "citizenship" expectations held of all employees. Examples of this include such things as maintaining current license, registration, or certification; attendance at any mandatory educational programs; participation in PI; customer satisfaction; teamwork; compliance with the dress code, time, and attendance requirements; organizational core values; etc. The job description should reflect both the primary responsibilities (essential functions) of the job and performance expectations that must be met to ensure continued employment.

competency   **employee**   **performance**

Chapter Four

The scale is used to illustrate the concepts of competency and performance. The goal is to have employees that are both competent (can carry out the primary responsibilities of their job) and who are good corporate citizens (adhere to organizational expectations of all employees). Leaders strive for a balance between the two concepts, thus ensuring safe, quality patient care and employees who adhere to the policies, respect each other, and demonstrate the mission, vision, ideals, and philosophy of the organization.

What do Joint Commission surveyors expect?

TJC surveyors evaluate the competency validation process by:

- Interviewing staff, often focusing on age-appropriate and population-appropriate aspects of care

- Observing delivery of care, including whether staff provide age-appropriate and population-appropriate care

- Conducting the competency assessment process review, in which they familiarize themselves with the organization's process for orientation, performance review, and competency validation (including its process for evaluating the delivery of age-appropriate and population-appropriate care)

- Reviewing requested employee-specific materials for evidence of orientation, initial/at-hire competency validation, continuing education, and ongoing competency validation

The review of employee-specific materials is the critical component of this part of TJC surveys. It is during this review that surveyors look for evidence that the processes identified by organizational leaders actually occur as described. Surveyors will ask staff to pull specific employee HR files for their review. Surveyors will request the files of staff they encountered during their individual and system tracer activities. Although the term "employee file" is frequently used to describe the location where the requested data are found, it may actually be a misnomer. The surveyors actually want to view the employee's materials related to orientation and competency validation, and these are frequently not found in the employee's HR file at all. They may be located in a variety of places, rather than one, including the department/unit where the employee works, the education department, with the employee's preceptor, with the agency from which the employee comes, and in the HR department. Regardless of where the data are ordinarily stored, when data are requested for viewing by TJC surveyors, staff members should assemble them quickly and present them to the surveyor.

Surveyors look for the following:

- Current job description

- Evidence of orientation, if hired in the last three years

- Competency validation, both at the end of orientation and ongoing competency validation

- Completed performance review

- Evidence of primary source verification of current licensure/registration/certification, if required for the job (as a performance expectation)

- Continuing education

Surveyors review the following information, not necessarily in this order:

- The qualification section of the job description to compare it against the qualifications of the employee. They will review the material, noting evidence of whether the organization completed primary source verification of any license, registration, or certificate required by law in order for the individual to practice. This documentation must be present at the time the person is hired and prior to the expiration of the license, registration, or certificate (this is the surveyors' way of validating at-hire competency).

- Evidence of orientation to the hospital, to the position, and to the department to which the employee was hired.

- The agenda for hospital orientation to ensure the required material is presented.

- Evidence of competency validation at the end of orientation, including validation of competency to perform primary responsibilities that have an age-related or population-related aspect to them, if applicable to the job.

- Ongoing competency assessment, including validation of the ability to perform completely the responsibilities that have an age-related/population-related aspect to them.

- Education records to determine whether the employee has completed competency-maintenance activities (for example, training, inservice education, seminars, etc.) that address the patient age groups and population groups identified in the job description as being the recipients of care, treatment, or service.

- Performance evaluations to ensure that leaders complete them with the frequency established in organizational policy and that they address the employee's ability to meet performance expectations stated in his or her job description (for example, adherence to organizationwide and departmental policies, professional standards, etc.).

Surveyors expect a competency validation process that includes all employees, not just those in clinical positions. They expect to see a process that validates the ability of staff members to provide care, treatment, or services to patients of different ages and different population groups, and to do this in a way that is appropriate to the ages and populations of the patients to whom they provide the care, treatment, or service. Age-specific competency validation should reflect the actual care given, through methods beyond testing just growth and development. Generalized approaches to validating age-appropriate care concepts, with no clear delineation of what this care actually entails or how it actually differs for the various age groups or populations, are no longer sufficient. Surveyors expect to see the methodology used to validate competency and not place a check mark next to the competency or state that the employee provides age-appropriate care without supporting evidence.

Chapter Five

What are validation methodologies?

What are validation methodologies?

Facilities can use a variety of techniques or methods to validate competency. These techniques or methods used to evaluate employees' abilities to carry out the primary responsibilities of the job are called validation methodologies. Validation methodologies evaluate employees' abilities, knowledge, and skills, and employees' application of required job skills, tasks, and activities to their actual performance. There are at least nine different validation methodologies, each of which is appropriate for use in verifying certain types of skills. These methodologies include the following:

- Post-test
- Return demonstration/observation of work
- Case study/discussion group
- Exemplar
- Peer review
- Self-assessment
- Presentation
- Simulation/drill
- Performance improvement (PI) monitoring and evaluation indicators

This chapter will define each methodology and show how organizations apply it to the validation process.

What to validate

Before using any of the validation methodologies listed above, the leader must identify what he or she is going to validate. All jobs require the performance of specific activities or tasks. These tasks may be:

- Psychomotor tasks
- Cognitive tasks
- Interpersonal tasks

Chapter Five

These tasks or activities are job skills. To perform the job skills well, individuals must possess certain knowledge, abilities, and skills. The combination of knowledge, abilities, and skills for a particular job is called a skill set.

The job description should state the activities an employee will be expected to perform and the skill set required to perform the job competently. Examples of specific job tasks and activities include:

- Registering a patient
- Administering medications
- Preparing meals
- Coding medical records
- Cleaning rooms
- Maintaining the boilers
- Leading a team
- Preparing the budget
- Strategic planning

It is each unit or department leader's responsibility to identify the skill set for each job in his or her unit or department and to incorporate that skill set into the job description. Because employees are more familiar with their jobs than anyone else, leaders should include employees in this process.

What are dimensions of a job skill?

Validation methodologies are the means the organization uses to ensure that each employee is competent in performing the skill set identified in his or her job description. Each methodology is unique and should focus on assessing specific aspects of skills, called dimensions. The three dimensions of skills are: critical thinking, interpersonal, and technical. Many jobs require competency in more than one of these dimensions.

The critical-thinking dimension is the ability to use information or knowledge. It involves more than just retaining facts; it demonstrates the employee's ability to apply knowledge to an actual situation. Critical thinking includes skills such as:

- Problem solving
- Time management
- Planning
- Fiscal responsibility
- Clinical reasoning
- Change management

The interpersonal dimension is the ability to work with others and includes skills and abilities such as:

- Communication
- Customer service
- Conflict management
- Working as a member of a team
- Understanding diversity

The technical dimension involves both possessing knowledge about a particular topic and the ability to perform fine and gross motor functions. It includes:

- Cognitive abilities
- Knowledge (for example, learned facts)
- Psychomotor ability (for example, the ability to operate equipment or perform physical tasks)
- Technical understanding (for example, how to program a computer)

Selecting the appropriate validation methodology

When validating a job skill, it is important to validate all applicable dimensions of the job, and to match the appropriate dimension(s) with the right methodology. If the leader does not validate all applicable dimensions of each skill, he or she might neglect important aspects of the job. Before selecting a validation methodology, the leader should decide which dimension(s) of the skill, task, or activity are important to validate. He or she might need to communicate with staff in the education or HR department before making this decision. Figure 5.1 identifies which methodologies are best suited to each skill dimension.

Figure 5.1 — Validation methodologies and the dimensions of competency they measure

Methodology	Technical	Critical thinking	Interpersonal
Post-test	x		
Demonstration/observation	x		
Case studies/discussion group	x	x	x
Exemplar		x	x
Peer review		x	x
Self-assessment		x	
Presentation	x	x	x
Simulation drill	x	x	x
PI monitoring	x	x	x

What are validation methodologies?

Many organizations do not assess job skills effectively or thoroughly because they often use only a one-dimensional competency validation process, or they apply an inappropriate validation methodology to the dimension they are validating. For example, a validation process that assesses only an employee's possession of certain knowledge will do little to tell a leader about the employee's ability to communicate with diverse populations. An example might be a nurse who is an expert in performing psychomotor tasks but alienates all coworkers and who is frequently described by patients and coworkers as "uncaring."

If communication is an important aspect of the employee's job, the leader should select a method to validate this competency. Similarly, if the ability to perform technical tasks or functions is important, the selected validation method should validate this ability rather than communication skills.

Because almost every job requires working with others, knowledge of how to perform the job, and the ability to perform certain tasks, organizations should use a variety of methodologies to assess competency. We have probably all seen individuals who perform tasks well technically but fail in more interpersonal areas. To avoid such a scenario, it is best to assess the cognitive and interpersonal dimensions of the job in conjunction with the technical dimension. A three-dimensional approach results in a three-dimensional view of the employee's skill set and performance of primary responsibilities.

The nine methodologies

Post-test

A post-test is a tool used after an educational session to evaluate how much information from the session an employee has retained. Although some people might refer to post-tests simply as tests, the healthcare industry prefers the term post-test. Post-tests are used in healthcare settings in much the same way as tests administered in academic settings evaluate a person's ability to repeat facts to demonstrate knowledge gained. If you would like to evaluate an employee's retention of newly learned facts, then a post-test is an appropriate methodology to use.

Post-tests can take the form of written tests, games (for example, bingo or *Jeopardy!*), or puzzles and are administered after an employee has received some sort of education related to his or her job. The educational material can be administered via a self-instructional packet, a live lecture, an audio- or videotape, or the reading of journal articles or books. As you can see from Figure 5.1, post-tests are intended to validate the technical dimension of a skill, task, or activity. It is the technical dimension that includes cognitive abilities or the ability to "know" something.

Return demonstration/observation of work

In return demonstration, a leader asks an employee to show how he or she performs a skill or task after the employee has learned the correct technique. This validation methodology is referred to as "return demonstration" because the employee demonstrates the technique after "receiving" education, meaning he or she "returns" the knowledge via the demonstration. The employee's education can be in the form of listening to a lecture or demonstration by an expert, reviewing a written procedure, completing a self-instructional packet or training manual, or viewing a training video. The employee can demonstrate his or her new knowledge in the actual work environment or in a simulated environment such as a skills lab or computer lab.

Observation of work is a technique leaders use to review an employee's actual work. This technique is best used for an employee who produces something in the process of doing his or her job, such as creating a spreadsheet, developing a budget, making a cabinet, writing a report, making a bed, sending a message via e-mail, etc.

Both return demonstration and observation of work assess psychomotor activity and require the leader to develop and use a checklist—often called a skills checklist—that serves as a standard or guideline for technical performance. The checklist should delineate the critical elements the leader expects to see, either in the return demonstration or during observation. The leader marks "yes" or "no" beside each of the critical elements on the checklist to validate which skills, tasks, and activities the employee performed correctly.

Case study/discussion group

Case studies and discussion groups are techniques for evaluating critical thinking and problem solving (critical-thinking dimension) and interpersonal dynamics (interpersonal dimension). Discussion groups are simply case studies discussed in a group setting—employees converse with each other and a facilitator rather than explore a scenario alone. In a discussion group, the facilitator both guides the group participants in discussion and validates competency. The facilitator listens for evidence of critical-thinking and problem-solving skills as staff members discuss the actions they would take and the rationales for their decisions.

In both case studies and discussion groups, the leader or facilitator presents the employees with a familiar work scenario. The employees are then asked to discuss:

- The decisions they would make or the action(s) they would take if faced with the same scenario

WHAT ARE VALIDATION METHODOLOGIES?

- Their rationales for the action(s) they selected

- Why they did not choose other courses of action

This technique allows employees the option to say that they would do nothing in the given situation, as the option of no action taken is always a possibility and is sometimes the most appropriate option.

In both validation methodologies, an "expert" in the area being validated must first determine the issues that should surface in the discussion of possible courses of action and the ideas that should frame the decision-making. These ideas could come from current scientific knowledge/law/organizational policy/regulatory directives/professional standards. The leader or facilitator—either the unit or department leader, or an outside facilitator chosen for his or her expert knowledge and ability to lead a discussion group—listens for these key issues and ideas in each employee's framing of the scenario and exploration of available courses of action. Rather than listen for one correct course of action, the leader or facilitator assesses each employee's ability to apply knowledge, think critically, and solve problems.

This is the primary way in which the case study/discussion group technique differs from a post-test. In a post-test there is only one correct answer for each question, but there are several possible courses of action with the case study/discussion group technique. The challenge for the employee is to identify all possible options and choose one course of action.

The case-study/discussion group methodology validates cognitive ability and critical thinking, and even age-specific cognitive ability and critical thinking. It also can validate critical thinking and interpersonal relations (see the example for the nonclinical setting that follows).

Case studies and discussion groups can be used in both clinical and nonclinical settings. In a clinical setting, case studies and discussion groups can validate age-specific cognitive ability and critical thinking. When performing such a validation, the leader or facilitator asks staff members several questions to validate their knowledge of the patient's disease process and their ability to apply this knowledge to the scenario and make a clinical assessment. The facilitator then asks participants to choose a course of action based on their clinical assessment and to give the rationale for their chosen course of action. Participants must then apply the same findings to a patient in a different age group.

In a nonclinical scenario, case studies and discussion groups can validate critical thinking and interpersonal relations. For example, they might be used to validate the competency of the registration clerks in both the registration process and in customer service.

Exemplar

An exemplar is essentially a case study in reverse. In a case study, the leader provides staff members with a scenario and then looks for certain competencies; in an exemplar, the leader identifies the competency that is being assessed and asks employees to discuss actual events in which they demonstrated competency. Employees then discuss their rationales for the actions they took and how their actions support organizational policy, professional standards, current knowledge in the field being discussed, etc. Like the case study/discussion group methodology, this methodology is useful in evaluating all three dimensions of a skill, task, or activity.

Peer review

In peer review, the leader assesses employee competency by obtaining the input of others who perform the same job. The peer review tool is typically a written form composed of a short series of statements containing attributes or behaviors consistent with organizational policy, standards, etc. Reviewers—others who perform the same job—complete the form, rating the employee on each statement using a Likert scale (a rating scale ranging from a response of five, indicating strong agreement, to a response of one, indicating strong disagreement) or true/false options.

The peer-review tool is usually developed by someone in the HR or education departments who is knowledgeable about test construction. The person constructing the evaluation tool must have input from individuals recognized as experts in the competency being evaluated. Their evaluation is based on observation of their peer interacting with others or on their own personal experiences with their peer. The individuals participating in peer review are frequently selected for this activity by the leader of the employee being evaluated. If there are few individuals performing a certain job, the leader might ask all of them to participate in a peer review of an individual.

Self-assessment

Self-assessment is one of the most frequently used validation methodologies, but it is also the most misused methodology. Although self-assessment is intended to assess the critical-thinking dimension of job skills, it is frequently used to validate psychomotor skills. For example, employees are frequently asked to complete self-assessments of their abilities to use various pieces of equipment normally encountered in performing their jobs. Because using equipment is a psychomotor skill, an assessment tool designed to assess psychomotor skills, such as demonstration or observation of actual work, would be appropriate for evaluating this competency. Self-assessment is not appropriate, as it does not evaluate psychomotor skills.

Self-assessment is a means for employees to assess their own assumptions about the work they do and the people they encounter while doing their jobs. Unlike other methodologies, self-assessment cannot be used independently to validate a competency. Its main purpose is to help employees recognize their own beliefs and values, and how those beliefs might affect the decisions employees make in doing their jobs.

In a typical self-assessment, an employee completes a written exercise that his or her leader has developed. This exercise might be a series of statements with which the employee agrees or disagrees, short statements with blanks that need to be filled in, or some other test instrument.

Unlike the tools previously discussed, self-assessment is intended to identify the employee's beliefs and values. Therefore, it relies upon the employee's self-awareness. As a result of discussing their beliefs and values with their leaders, employees can identify how their beliefs and values might be impediments to properly completing job skills, tasks, or activities. The actual impediment to competency might be that an employee's value system is incongruent with organizational policy. Unless the organization identifies and addresses this incongruence, the employee will continue to perform in a manner that is inconsistent with the organization's established standards.

For example, an individual who believes that children under the age of two do not experience pain—or that, if they do experience pain, they do not remember it—will often follow a different course of action when performing painful procedures than a person who believes that those same children do experience pain. Approaches to pain management might also differ, depending on the person's beliefs about childhood pain.

Self-assessment can be used in conjunction with peer review to identify incongruence between an individual's beliefs and values, and a peer's observations of how the person actually behaves in a situation.

Presentation

A presentations is appropriate to use when validating someone's cognitive, technical-understanding, and critical-thinking abilities. Leaders can use presentations to evaluate an employee's mastery of new knowledge. In this technique, an employee agrees to present to other employees the new knowledge he or she has learned through a seminar, individual readings, or some other educational endeavor. An expert on the subject of the presentation should be present to evaluate the employee's knowledge. The expert validating the employee's knowledge should record his or her assessment of the employee, then send the assessment to the person's department/unit leader. The leader will then use it to validate competency. Leaders might wish to combine this technique with another methodology that would evaluate the competency of employees attending the presentation.

Simulation/drill

TJC requires that healthcare organizations conduct a variety of drills and simulations. These drills include fire, disaster, infant and pediatric abduction, and hazardous spills. Some organizations choose to conduct additional simulations, such as mock codes, internal disasters, and hazardous spill clean-up.

All drills offer an opportunity to validate competency without the leader having to do any additional work. If the evaluation forms completed after the drill or simulation can be designed to identify individual behavior, not just to identify employees as a group (e.g., "the staff in the laboratory"), the critique form can serve as evidence of competency. This might also serve as an effective complement to the annual review of the environment-of-care plans that OSHA requires, because it demonstrates an employee's actual behavior rather than his or her mere retention of facts.

PI monitoring

Leaders can assess competency while gathering data for use in PI. It is likely that there are existing PI indicators that can assess interpersonal competencies (e.g., patient satisfaction surveys), critical-thinking competencies (e.g., adequacy of pain control), and technical competencies (e.g., user errors associated with biomedical equipment). Other than developing a tool to identify the desired behaviors that can be individualized to employees, leaders can simultaneously validate a competency and complete a required activity without having to do any additional work.

Rules and tools

No method can be used to validate competency without an identified way staff members are to perform the activity (the rule) and without tools developed to allow the activity/responsibility to be assessed. Rules are the written policy, procedure, protocol, guideline, etc., that specify how something is to be done. The tool(s) used to validate competency reflect the critical steps/concepts found in the rule. When more than one discipline performs the same activity (for example, venipuncture), the rules for how it is to be done, including how it should be done differently for patients of different ages, and the tool(s) used to validate competency of the various staff members performing this activity, should be the same. In this way, consistency in performance of an activity will be realized, regardless of which staff members actually perform the activity. Without rules (policies, procedures, protocols, etc.) that uniformly apply to all staff members performing an activity and validation tools reflective of the critical steps of the rule used to validate competency of all staff performing an activity, there can be variation in practice and differing patient experiences.

Common pitfalls

Perhaps because of familiarity or ease of use, many leaders rely almost exclusively on three methodologies to validate a competency: post-test, observation/demonstration, and self-assessment. Such reliance on these three methods might prevent a complete assessment of a competency and actually waste time by providing little useful information. The organization creates more work for leaders than necessary, and competency validation becomes yet another task for the leader to complete, often with no tangible benefit for the organization or to the employee.

To save time and avoid unnecessary work, leaders should look for every opportunity to use existing data to provide information about staff competency. Examples of existing data include simulations, drills, and PI reports.

Applying the nine methodologies: A hypothetical case study

The examples that follow illustrate how an organization might apply the nine validation methodologies or techniques to validate employee competency in a given situation. The scenario appears first, followed by descriptions of how the organization in the example could use each of the nine methodologies.

A clinic has decided to open a pediatric diabetes program. While the clinic already has a diabetes program, the pediatric diabetic patients have been receiving care in the same setting and from the same staff as have adult patients. Parent dissatisfaction with the adult diabetes program, coupled with data indicating a fourfold increase in the number of children diagnosed with diabetes, indicated the need for this program. The new program will be the pilot site for the new patient registration computer program, and new glucose monitoring devices will be used in the setting. The majority of the clinical staff in the new program transferred from the adult site.

Post-test
The clinic uses modules to educate the large number of clinical employees selected to work in the new pediatric program. These modules contain information on the pathophysiology of diabetes, including the different signs of onset based on the age at which the disease manifests itself,

and new treatment options proving effective for adolescent diabetics. The self-learning module also outlines normal glucose values for the various age groups making up the program's patient population. After reading the packet, each staff member takes an individual written post-test comprising 20 multiple choice and true/false questions. The clinic uses the post-tests to evaluate the staff's retention of the facts included in the self-instructional packet. Lastly, all staff participate in a *Jeopardy!*-based game, with answers coming from the information in the modules.

Return demonstration/observation of work
Because the clinic's new pediatric diabetes program utilizes new glucose monitors, staff must learn how to use them. The manufacturer supplies an educator to discuss the features of the new monitors and demonstrate how to use them. The staff members then complete a crossword puzzle, with the questions coming from the educator's presentation. If a staff member completes at least 85% of the puzzle correctly, he or she then demonstrates to the educator the proper technique for using the monitor. The educator completes a checklist for each staff member, observing the performance of the critical elements of the procedure. In this example, the organization uses a post-test (the crossword puzzle) to assess cognitive ability and a return demonstration (the staff member's demonstration of proper technique) to assess technical understanding and psychomotor skill.

While clinical staff members are receiving information and validating competency in the use of the new glucose monitors, registration staff are shown how to use the new computer system to register patients. Observation of actual work (registration of patients when the clinic opens) will be utilized to validate staff competency.

Case study/discussion group
The clinic leader determines that customer service is a competency that all staff should have. The leader presents the following scenario to registration staff:

A tired and angry parent is attempting to register a child in the clinic, while still caring for three other children who are all under the age of five.

Staff members discuss how they might be of service to the parent while completing the registration process. By exploring possible courses of action in this scenario, the clinic's standards of customer service can be reinforced. The group leader listens for customer service principles during staff discussion, filing a notation on each employee in his or her personnel file.

Exemplar

One goal of the new pediatric diabetes program is to provide quality customer service. An environmental service employee tells his leader about a situation that just occurred in which the employee demonstrated customer service by stopping to assist a lost, frustrated, and angry parent. Although such assistance is not normally part of the employee's job, the leader can use the employee's rationale for why the action he took supports the organizational goal, and the example itself, to validate the employee's critical thinking and interpersonal dimensions of his job.

Peer review

The clinic leader develops a peer review tool. Each statement is followed by a five-point rating scale, with five indicating "always" and one indicating "never." The peer review tool is intended for use with all staff working in the new pediatric program. Employees in similar job groups complete the tool, indicating their observations of the other employee(s) being validated. Upon completion, employees return the tool to the leader so that he or she can review the responses.

Self-assessment

Most of the clinic's registration clerks have successfully transitioned to the new registration process, but a few have not. The leader knows that those who have not successfully transitioned do possess the technical skills to perform the job skills because he or she validated their abilities using observation of actual work. All staff members complete self-assessments regarding the management of change, and the leader finds that staff members who are not successfully using the new computer system view the new registration process simply as a way to reduce the number of registration clerks. The leader avoids wasting time reeducating the employees in how to use the new computer program, addressing instead their fear of change.

Presentation

The clinic sends an employee from environmental services and another from registration to a two-day seminar on customer service. When they return, they agree to share with other staff members in the clinic what they learned in the seminar. In this way, all staff members have access to the knowledge these two employees have gained. In addition, giving the presentation validates competency for the two presenters. The clinic leader develops an evaluation tool, including the major points of customer service the two employees should include in their presentation.

In addition to validating the technical competency of the two presenters, the leader decides to use the presentation as an opportunity to validate the technical competency of the attendees. The leader develops a short post-test, with content assistance from the two presenters. Following the presentation, all attendees complete the post-test.

Simulation drill

To meet TJC requirements, the clinic must hold at least one fire drill per year. The leader sees the fire drill as an opportunity to validate competency of all staff members working during the drill. The leader designs a critique form to validate staff members' competency in both the technical and critical-thinking dimensions of this life-safety competency. This form identifies the critical steps staff members must follow according to the clinic's fire plan. To validate knowledge, staff members have watched a video on fire response in clinics and have taken a post-test. All staff working during the drill must verbalize the steps they would take during an actual fire, locate the closest pull box and fire extinguisher, and determine whether they would first remove patients or records from the fire. The leader selects observers to assist in this competency validation, so that competency can be verified for all staff. Observers complete a competency validation form for each employee.

PI monitoring

The clinic leader selects as a PI indicator the quality of the documentation that clinical staff members make in the patient record. Instead of simply reviewing the records for completeness, the leader decides to use this activity to validate the competency of individual staff members. The review form used for this evaluation contains not only the critical elements of a complete record entry, as specified in clinic policy, but also a place to record the name(s) of individual staff members making the entry. If documentation is complete, it serves as evidence of technical competency.

Chapter six

Ongoing measure of core competency

Ongoing measure of core competency

The previous chapters have discussed the basics of competency, establishing competency programs, validating competency, and validation methodologies. You now have the knowledge and tools to take competency to the next level: that of establishing an ongoing measure of core competency.

"Data" is defined by the 2008 Hospital Accreditation Standards Glossary as "uninterpreted observations or facts." "Aggregate data" is a term used to define the process of using data that are rolled up from a smaller unit to show the data in summary. Using such aggregate data to measure ongoing core competency will be the string that ties the pieces of your competency program together.

In an effort to comply with regulations, adhere to "best practices," and operationalize performance improvement programs, healthcare facilities collect copious amounts of data. Data that are trended, analyzed, and aggregated can be valuable to managers in assessing ongoing competency. Aggregate data are routinely collected for infection control, risk management, and safety. Interpreting the data and aggregating the information over time to validate ongoing competency can streamline the evaluation process and bring relevancy to the competency assessment program.

Using data to measure competency

Organizations can use data for numerous purposes. For purposes of this discussion, we will look at data that are designed to identify educational opportunities and to validate competency.

There are a number of typical categories of data that organizations use in their competency validation programs.

Risk:

- Incident reports
- Patient injury
- Medication errors
- Risk-management reports
- Failure modes and effects analysis
- Sentinel events

Outcome:

- Code/RRT statistics
- Hospital-acquired infection reports
- Readmission reports
- Core measure data

Satisfaction/complaint:

- Patient
- Employee
- Physician

Environment of care:

- Equipment management
- Disaster preparedness
- User error reports
- Fire safety
- Fire responsiveness
- Role in education and protection of patient and staff

Management of HR:

- Cross-training modules
- Past performance and competency evaluations
- Employee suggestions/complaints

Data mining

Data mining, defined as the extraction of hidden predictive information that exists in large databases, is a powerful and relatively new technology with tremendous potential that can help corporations to focus on the most important information in their data storage.

Healthcare organizations can learn from industry how to "mine" for the information that can help them become more proactive by looking at hidden trends and patterns that exist outside of normal expectations. Data-mining techniques can be implemented as a means to better understand the meaning behind the numbers.

Anomalous data are made up of information that results from errors or unusual events. For example, keying errors in data entry may obscure important information related to medication errors.

Outlier data may have been overlooked in the past. These should be examined more closely as they may carry important information related to time of event, etc.

Using aggregate data and data-mining techniques to identify competency needs

Data that have been aggregated (i.e., summarized) over time, relating to competency of certain procedures, processes, etc., can be a valuable tool to identify areas in which staff members need further improvement before competency can be validated. There are many examples of ways in which organizations use aggregate data in their competency validation program.

Research has shown that medication errors can occur due to a number of varying causes:

- Insufficient or incorrect information collected about the patient related to weight, allergies, comorbidities, and lab results
- Lack of up-to-date information about the medication
- Inappropriate use of abbreviations
- Legibility issues
- Inadequate or mislabeled medications
- Interruptions and other distractions

Medication error reporting serves as a good example of how to integrate aggregate data into your competency program based on previously known data categories.

Chapter six

Medication error reports may be collected and categorized using four major elements:

- Ordering
- Transcription
- Administration
- Documentation

Data may reveal that medication errors/administration errors more frequently than other elements.

Aggregated data that have been summarized over time and analyzed even further to indicate the type of administration and to be individualized by the employee may tell you more.

Aggregated data displayed in such a manner as in Figure 6.1 clearly indicate an educational opportunity for employee #231 related to medication administration with a focus on missed and incorrect dose errors.

Data mining, if available, may be able to provide further drill-down in the data elements to reveal, for example, that the drop-down codes for certain after-hour medications were similar for certain medications. The organization learns that keystroke error entries were frequently made by this employee; thus the error is even further defined and education needs can be determined.

Using aggregated data appropriately allows department managers or organization leaders the ability to identify learning needs for specific employees. Data in general can assist with developing unit-specific goals related to education. See Figure 6.2 for an example.

Leaders and managers must be given the skills and data-collection tools necessary to aggregate, analyze, and act appropriately when data reveal opportunities for staff education and improvement in patient care.

Figure 6.1 — Analyzing medication error data

Ordering	3
Transcribing	17
Administration	24
Documentation	8

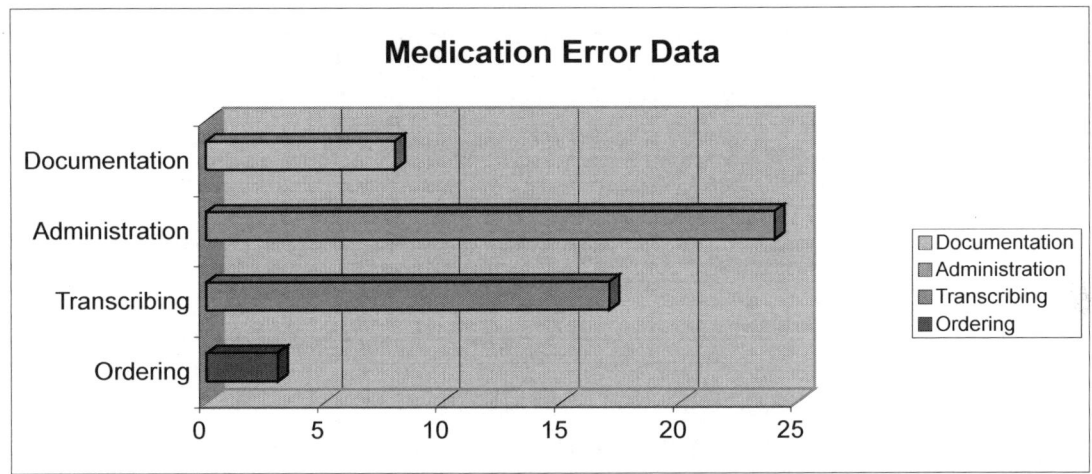

Employee #	675	231	643	943
Wrong patient	0	1	0	2
Incorrect route	1	2	0	1
Incorrect dose	1	3	0	3
Missed dose (based on policy)	4	7	2	2

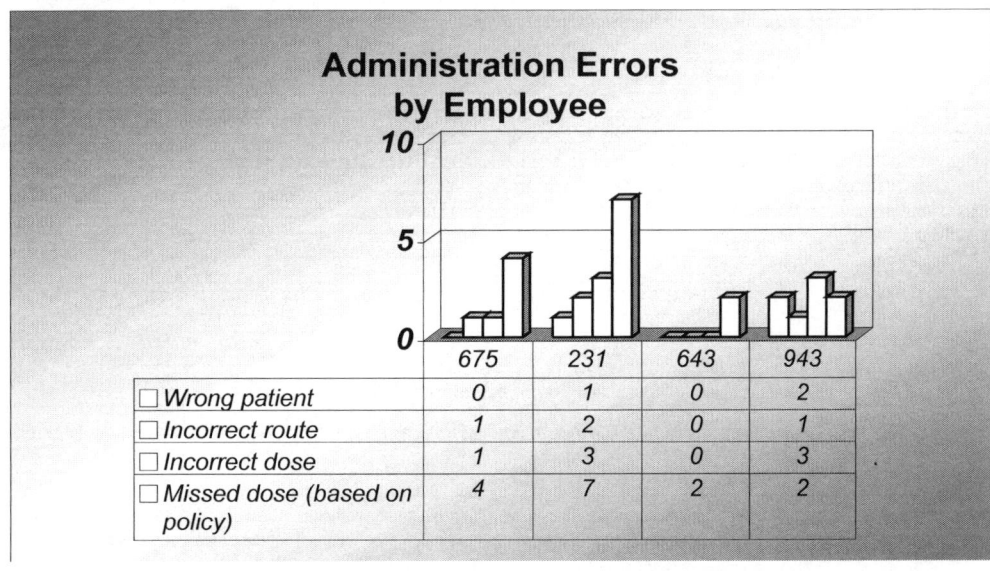

Figure 6.2 — Aggregated medication error data

Medication administration errors for the past year by employee #	Narcotic	Floor stock	Override (automated dispensing)	After-hour pharmacy access
456	0	2	0	1
754	1	0	1	0
821	2	1	3	6
905	0	0	0	0
630	0	1	1	1

Using aggregate data to validate competency

Data can be used to demonstrate the need for additional education, knowledge, practice, etc., in much the same way that they can be used to demonstrate and validate competency of personnel. As we have previously discussed, data are collected for many purposes. Healthcare organizations are developing strategies that define the potential purpose and use of data. Data that may represent the potential to validate competency must be collected.

Practitioner-specific data that are aggregated over time are a powerful tool in validating competency. Collecting, verifying, and summarizing the data ensures that the information will be viewed as an accurate reflection of the competency of the individual.

Establish a consistent method of data collection. All personnel involved in the data collection must be trained and understand the importance of collecting data using the same methodology. For example, "complete" may have different meanings to different people. Define all data collection points and parameters to ensure validity. Policies and procedures that are current and accurately reflect practice can serve as data collection guides.

Performance data, when aggregated by trained individuals, allow staff to "rate" their competency compared to their peers. Displaying practitioner-specific, aggregated data as benchmarks of performance and competency can enhance a learning and professional growth environment (See Figure 6.3). Using aggregated data to validate competency can be rewarding. Providing your staff with an accurate assessment of their competency, free of subjectivity, results in assessments that are clearly stated, detailed, and specific, and can provide a foundation for growth and improvement.

Figure 6.3 — Section from pharmacist competency assessment

Date	*Criteria*	Evaluation method
	Aliquots in syringes such as dexamethasone 1. Observe calculations 2. Observe admixture 3. Observe order entry	• Observation and review of documentation • Compliance with written policy and procedure
	Order entry of antibiotics such as Rocephin 1. Pharmacist choosing the correct predefined Rocephin/IV bag combination in the computer based on final drug concentration, for example, 25ml, 50ml, 100ml bag	• Observation and review of documentation • Compliance with written policy and procedure
	TPN order entry and admixture of an adult nonstandard TPN 1. Observe calculations 2. Observe admixture 3. Observe order entry	• Observation and review of documentation • Compliance with written policy and procedure
	Pharmacokinetic calculations, order entry, admixture, and labeling of vancomycin IV doses based on reduced renal clearance, for example, dose/schedule modification	• Observation and review of documentation • Compliance with written policy and procedure
	Gentamicin protocol dosing regimen based on advanced age/ reduced renal clearance	• Observation and review of documentation • Compliance with written policy and procedure

Source: Developed by Chanda Flynn, RN, MSN, CEN, assistant chief nursing officer, Mary Black Health System, Spartanburg, SC, with input from Judd Seay and Glenda Thackston

Chapter seven

The competency validation process

The competency validation process

'Putting the pieces together'

Case study by Aultman Hospital, Canton, OH

As a large tertiary hospital, we struggled to clearly understand not only what was needed to meet the Joint Commission's competency standards but more importantly how we could validate and feel confident that our bedside caregivers were competent. After much discussion, consultation from The Greeley Company, research, and education, we believe we have found a process that is clearly understood by not only the leaders in our organization but by the managers and bedside caregivers as well. We have structured our program into four steps as described below. Please see Figure 7.1 for a depiction of the process.

Step 1: Initial competency validation at time of hire

This step includes the initial interview completed by Human Resources (HR); reference and background checks; primary source license validation, if applicable; and matching the applicant to the job qualifications. This step is most likely already in place within your organization. Please see Figure 7.2.

Step 2: Orientation—the education process

Before discussion of this step occurs, it's important to recognize that education does not prove competency. This concept was new to many of our managers and required in-depth discussions and a mutual understanding before we could move forward with the new process. The standards require that competency must be validated at the conclusion of orientation.

To better understand how this concept applies, ask yourself the following question: What are the expectations of a new bedside caregiver at the conclusion of orientation? More than likely, your answer will be that the caregiver can perform the core competencies of the job. This is central to understanding competency validation at the conclusion of orientation.

Chapter Seven

Figure 7.1 — Competency validation process

Step 1: Initial competency validation at time of hire

- Interview
- References
- Primary source license validation
- Job qualification validation

Step 2: Orientation—The education process

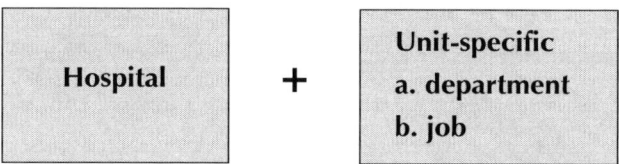

Validation of core competencies at conclusion of orientation
(Core competencies identified as age-related and validated as such)

Step 3: Ongoing competency validation

- Unit-specific
- Age-related
- Ongoing for a period of time (e.g., one year)
- Continuous fluid process (items can be added throughout year)
- Individualized

1. Mandated competencies (e.g., safety, NPSGs)
2. New/changed competencies
3. Low-volume/high-risk competencies
4. Problem-prone competencies (identified by aggregate data)

Step 4: Annual performance evaluation according to policy

Performance review to include organizational expectations

THE COMPETENCY VALIDATION PROCESS

Figure 7.2

Applicant worksheet

_____ Hospital

Name _____

Position applied for _____ Unit/department _____ Date applied _____

Initial interview date _____ Interviewed by _____

Date education verified _____

Verified with _____ at _____

with _____ at _____

Date license, registration, certification(s) verified _____

License as _____ verified with _____

Registration as _____ verified with _____

Certification verified with _____

Reference request form signed on _____ References requested on _____

Received on _____ from _____

on _____ from _____

on _____ from _____

Interview with _____ (unit/department leader)

scheduled for _____

Hire: ❑ Yes   ❑ No

Offer made (pending background check and employee health screening) on _____

Accepted   ❑ Yes   ❑ No

Criminal background check completed on _____

Urine drug screen completed on _____

Cleared by Employee Health on _____

Hospital orientation scheduled _____

Department orientation on _____

Signature _____ Date _____

COMPETENCY ASSESSMENT, THIRD EDITION

Orientation to the hospital is required and has three components. The first is orientation to the organization. The second is orientation to the unit/work area. The third is orientation to the job. Orientation length fluctuates depending on the job classification of each new hire. At the end of orientation to the job, validation of core competencies must be completed. In our organization, core competencies and job descriptions are used interchangeably. Figure 7.3 is the tool we developed for use in validating competency at the end of orientation for all RNs and for the unit-specific expectations for an RN in one of our critical care units. Figure 7.4 is for the registered radiologic technologist (RRT), and Figure 7.5 is for the security officer. The unit manager, using input from the preceptor and new employee, completes an evaluation documenting that the new employee is competent to perform the job duties. Since core competencies rarely change, they only need to be validated at the end of orientation unless there is a reason to revalidate due to some aggregate data source or cause for concern.

Step 3: Ongoing competency validation

The newest piece in our competency process was the implementation of an ongoing competency program. The ongoing competency program must be unit-specific, age-related, ongoing for a defined period of time (for example, one year), and a continuous, fluid process allowing new competencies to be added. The ongoing competency tool can be individualized for each employee. Key attributes include:

- Organization-mandated competencies such as safety
- Department-mandated competencies
- New or changed competencies
- Low-volume/high-risk competencies
- Problem-prone competencies as identified by aggregate data

Unit managers develop the ongoing competency assessment tool specific for their unit and patient population. Figure 7.6 represents those ongoing competencies an RN in one of the critical care units must validate within the year. Figure 7.7 represents this information for an RRT and Figure 7.8 for a security officer.

The tool may differ for each caregiver as needed in order to address individual variations and specific aggregate data concerns. The ongoing competency assessment tool is reviewed annually and revised for the following year. In addition, any new or changed competencies that were identified will be moved to the core competency/job description and will be included in future new employees' orientation to the job.

Step 4: Annual performance evaluation

The last step in the competency validation process is an annual performance appraisal/evaluation. In our organization, a decision was made to develop one tool that will be used for each employee during this review. The tool includes organizational expectations that each employee much fulfill. Figure 7.9 shows the tool we developed for this purpose.

Lessons learned

As we reflect on the process and review our progress, we have a few recommendations to share. First and foremost, solicit and gain the support of senior management before embarking on such a huge process change. Managers must be able to invest the time needed to create/revise core competencies as well as time to develop their ongoing unit-specific competencies for each job class. Managers need support in order to accomplish this task. Secondly, appoint an HR champion to coordinate the project. The champion needs to have a mechanism in place to track progress and the ability to work with unit managers in developing their tools. Finally, soliciting input from all stakeholders helps reduce the resistance to implementing a process change.

Feedback

To our surprise, the new competency validation process was received positively. Managers believe the new process reduces redundancy, is more relevant for evaluating caregivers, and simplifies the evaluation/performance appraisal process.

Chapter Seven

Figure 7.3 — Registered nurse job description

DRAFT

REGISTERED NURSE

Date:	Last revision date:
Employee name:	Job Title: REGISTERED NURSE
Employee number:	Reports to: Unit Director
Department:	
Signatures:	Select one of the following:
	____ Post-orientation competency assessment
Director: _____ Date: _____	____ Job evaluation
VP/AVP: _____ Date: _____	____ Annual performance evaluation
	____ New job

MISSION STATEMENT

BASIC PURPOSE OF THE JOB

The primary purpose of the Staff Nurse (Registered Nurse) is to provide clinical leadership of patient care, provide patient and family teaching, and work cooperatively with the healthcare team in maintaining standards of care within the framework of the Ohio Nurse Practice Act.

CONTACTS

Age of patient populations served *(Check all that apply)*

Neonates (1–30 days)	Adults (19 to 70 years)
Infants (30 days to 1 year)	Geriatric (>70 years)
Children (1–12 years)	
Adolescents (13–18 years)	No patient contact

Competency validation methods
- O = Observation/Demonstration
- PT = Posttest
- D = Drills
- PI = Performance improvement monitors

JOB REQUIREMENTS

- Graduate of an accredited school of nursing
- Current licensure to practice as a registered nurse in the state
- BLS certification
- Demonstrates proficiency in basic nursing care, knowledge, and skills
- Demonstrates knowledge of evidence-based practice

WORKING CONDITIONS

- Rotate shifts, works every other weekend and holidays as assigned
- Lunch and break periods are coordinated with other staff to maintain adequate coverage
- Hazardous exposure rating: 1
- Subject to frequent interruptions during performance of duties

Figure 7.3.xls

Figure 7.3: Registered nurse job description (cont.)

Core competencies/job description

Rating scale and definitions

2 = Consistently exceeds standards	Performs consistently; surpasses all established standards. Activities often contribute to improved or innovative work practices. This category is to be used for truly outstanding performance.
1 = Consistently meets/sometimes exceeds standards	Performance meets all established standards and sometimes exceeds them. Activities contribute to increased unit results. Employees consistently complete the work that is required and at times go beyond expectations.
0 = Developmental/needs improvement	Performance meets most but not all established standards. Activities sometimes contribute to unit results. This category is to be used for employees who must demonstrate improvement or more consistent performance and for employees still learning their job. Areas for improvement are included in the narrative.

Essential functions

Essential functions are those tasks, duties, and responsibilities that comprise the means of accomplishing the job's purpose and objectives. Essential functions are critical or fundamental to the performance of the job. They are the major functions that the person in the job is held accountable for. Following are the essential functions of the job, along with the corresponding performance standards:

Neonates	Infants	Children	Adolescents	Adults	Geriatrics	Validation method	Rating (0,1,2)

1. **Performs admissions assessment and reassessments as defined by policy.**
   a. Performs assessment in accordance with specific unit standards.
   b. Performs initial screening (i.e., pain, abuse, nutrition, skin, falls) and makes appropriate referrals.

Performance narrative

Neonates	Infants	Children	Adolescents	Adults	Geriatrics	Validation method	Rating (0,1,2)

2. **Formulates and updates plan of care according to policy.**
   a. Analyzes data to identify nursing care needs.
   b. Coordinates the care of patient from admission to discharge.
   c. Identifies nursing care needs and develops and updates individual plan of care based on analysis of data.
   d. Develops patient/family/significant other teaching and discharge plan as per unit standard.
   e. Assesses, plans, implements, and reevaluates the patient/family discharge needs from time of admission through discharge.

Performance narrative

CHAPTER SEVEN

Figure 7.3 **Registered nurse job description (cont.)**

Neonates	Infants	Children	Adolescents	Adults	Geriatrics	Validation method	Rating (0,1,2)

3. **Demonstrates the skills and judgment necessary to implement an evidence-based plan of care.**
   a. Administers medications following policies and procedures.
   b. Responds to clinical emergencies following policies and procedures.
   c. Demonstrates required skills and competencies in the use of equipment for care of the patient population common to the work area.
   d. Administers blood and blood products according to policies and procedures.
   e. Initiates and maintains IV access according to policies and procedures.
   f. Performs lab order entry according to policies and procedures.
   g. Utilizes Med Select/Pyxis according to policy.
   h. Utilizes patient identifiers.
   i. Able to transcribe orders following policies and procedures.

Performance narrative

4. **Identifies the patient's education needs and develops goals and educational objectives.**
   a. Consistently develops an individual education plan involving the family/significant other as defined by policy.
   b. Education plan is updated, revised, and reviewed in order to ensure consistent care from admission to discharge.
   c. Provides education according to patient needs.
   d. Evaluates education plan effectiveness and makes changes as appropriate.

Performance narrative

5. **Evaluates the patient's responses to care.**
   a. Performs reassessment according to policies and procedures.
   b. Analyzes data to identify ongoing nursing care needs.
   c. Modifies plan of care to meet patient's identified needs.

Performance narrative

Figure 7.3 — Registered nurse job description (cont.)

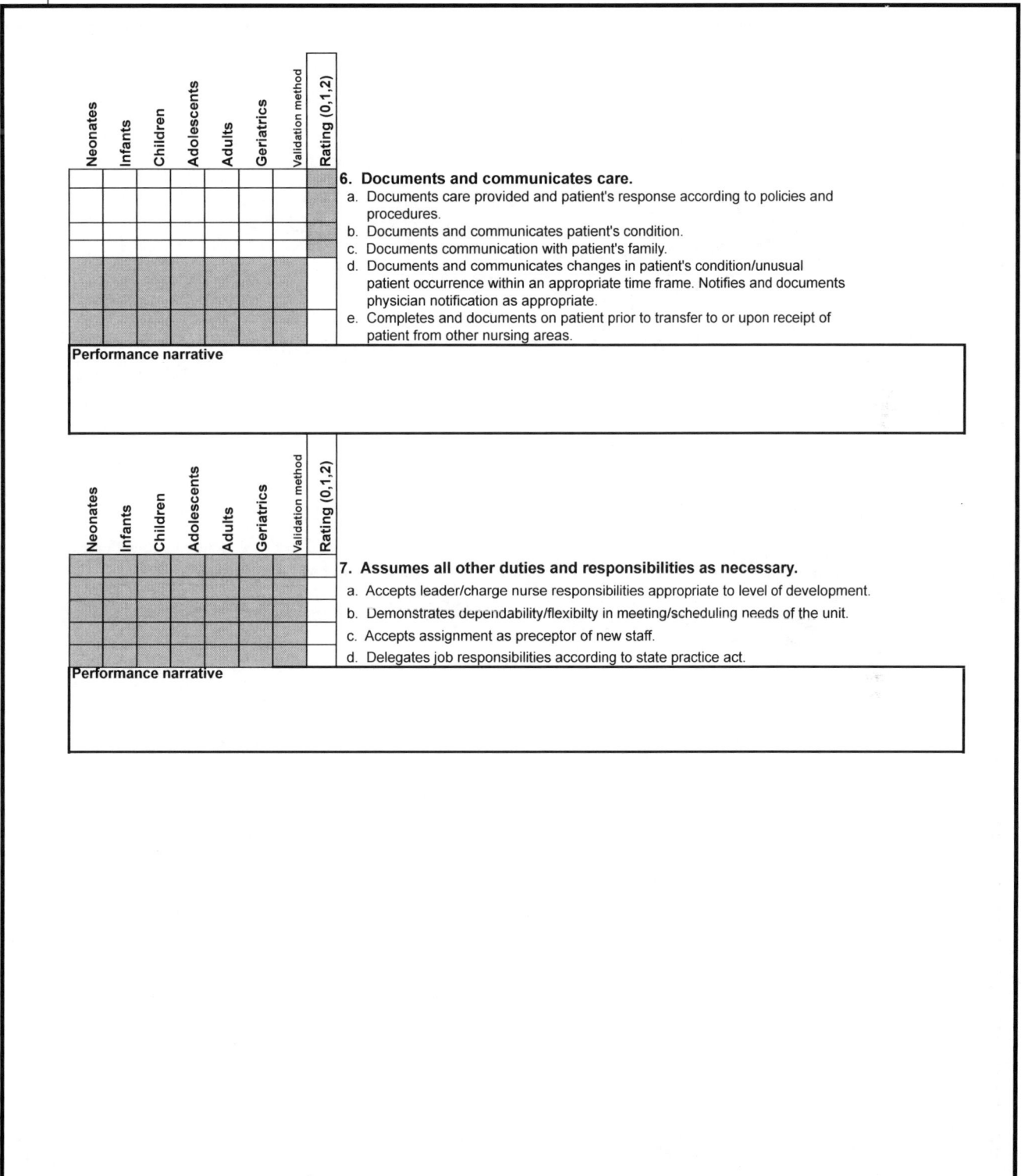

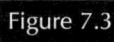

Registered nurse job description (cont.)

Unit-specific core competencies/job description
5 South—neuro-spine unit

Neonates	Infants	Children	Adolescents	Adults	Geriatrics	Validation method	Rating (0,1,2)	
								1. Demonstrates care of the patient with supportive devices.
								a. Cervical collar.
								b. Halo.
								c. TLSO.
								d. Lumbar.

Performance narrative

Neonates	Infants	Children	Adolescents	Adults	Geriatrics	Validation method	Rating (0,1,2)	
								2. Identifies and implements care specific to the neuro-spine patient.
								a. Able to perform a neurological assessment
								b. Recognizes and responds to changes in neurological assessment
								c. Recognizes and reacts to signs and symptoms of post-operative complications
								d. Demonstrates required competencies related to PCA/epidural pumps

Performance narrative

The competency validation process

Figure 7.3

Registered nurse job description (cont.)

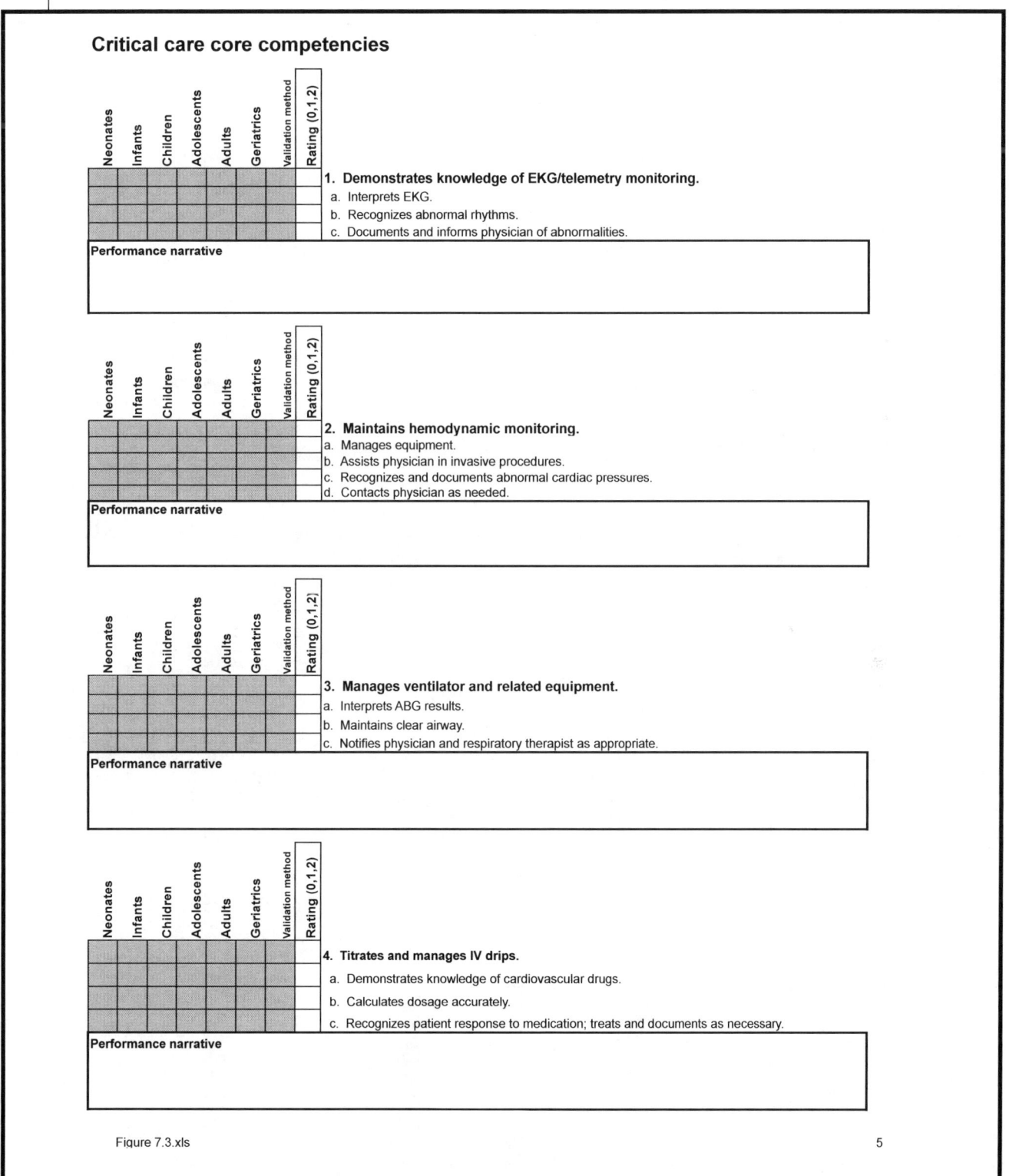

Figure 7.3.xls

Competency Assessment, Third Edition — **119**

Figure 7.4: Registered radiologic technologist job description

Job description and core performance standards

REVISED 8/04

REGISTERED RADIOLOGIC TECHNOLOGIST

Date:		Last revision date: 9/2004
Employee name:	Employee number:	Job title: REGISTERED RADIOLOGIC TECHNOLOGIST
Department:		Reports to: Unit Director

Signatures:

Select one of the following:
___ Post-orientation competency assessment
___ Other (as applicable)

Director: _____ Date: _____
VP/AVP: _____ Date: _____

BASIC PURPOSE OF THE JOB

Under the direction of a radiologist, the primary purpose of the radiologic technologist is to perform a variety of technical procedures requiring independent judgment and initiative to apply the prescribed diagnostic imaging equipment for the production of high-quality images.

CONTACTS

Age of Patient Populations Served *(Check all that apply)*

Neonates (1–30 days)	Adults (19–70 years)
Infants (30 days to 1 year)	Geriatric (>70 years)
Children (1–12 years)	
Adolescents (13–18 years)	No patient contact

WORKING CONDITIONS

- Work a variety of shifts 7 days a week including holiday rotation
- Subject to frequent interruptions during performance of duties
- Lunch periods and breaks are coordinated with other staff to maintain adequate unit coverage
- Adhere to hospital policies and procedures
- Fulfill core competency performance standards and organizational competency standards
- Considerable standing and walking
- Possible exposure to ionizing radiation
- Close contact with patients under mental and physical stress

JOB REQUIREMENTS

- Graduate of an accredited school of radiologic technology
- Current licensure to practice as a registered technologist in the state
- ARRT certification
- Demonstrates proficiency in basic patient care, knowledge, and skills
- Demonstrates knowledge on evidence-based practice

Competency validation methods
O = Observation/demonstration
PT = Post-test
D = Drills
PI = Performance improvement monitors

The Competency Validation Process

Figure 7.4: Registered radiologic technologist job description (cont.)

Core competencies/job description

Rating scale and definitions

2 = Consistently exceeds standards	Performance consistently surpasses all established standards. Activities often contribute to improved or innovative work practices. This category is to be used for truly outstanding performance.
1 = Consistently meets/sometimes exceeds standards	Performance meets all established standards and sometimes exceeds them. Activities contribute to increased unit results. Employees consistently complete the work that is required and at times go beyond expectations.
0 = Developmental/needs improvement	Performance meets most, but not all, established standards. Activities sometimes contribute to unit results. This category is to be used for employees who must demonstrate improvement or more consistent performance and for employees still learning their job. Areas for improvement are included in the narrative.

gray box indicates the activity is not age-related, white indicates age-specific

Essential functions

Essential functions are those tasks, duties, and responsibilities that comprise the means of accomplishing the job's purpose and objectives. Essential functions are critical or fundamental to the performance of the job. They are the major functions that the person in the job is held accountable for. Following are the essential functions of the job, along with the corresponding performance standards:

Neonates	Infants	Children	Adolescents	Adults	Geriatrics	Validation method	Rating (0,1,2)

1. Ensures that correct patient is having procedure performed as defined by policy.
   a. Name and medical record number verified 100% on all in-patients.
   b. Name and date of birth verified 100% on all out-patients.

Performance narrative

Neonates	Infants	Children	Adolescents	Adults	Geriatrics	Validation method	Rating (0,1,2)

2. Performs technical component of procedure according to protocols.
   a. Positions patient to obtain the desired results as prescribed.
   b. Measures, calculates, and selects proper electronic factors to produce high-quality images.
   c. Accurately performs procedures and adheres to established standards and protocols utilized in section.

Performance narrative

Chapter seven

Figure 7.4 — Registered radiologic technologist job description (cont.)

Neonates	Infants	Children	Adolescents	Adults	Geriatrics	Validation method	Rating (0,1,2)	
								3. Demonstrates the skills and judgment necessary to implement an evidence-based plan of care.
								a. Administers contrast following policies and procedures.
								b. Responds to clinical emergencies following policies and procedures.
								c. Demonstrates required skills and competencies in the use of equipment for care of the patient population common to the work area.

Performance narrative

Neonates	Infants	Children	Adolescents	Adults	Geriatrics	Validation method	Rating (0,1,2)	
								4. Identifies the patient's education needs.
								a. Consistently provides a simple explanation of procedures to patient/family.

Performance narrative

Neonates	Infants	Children	Adolescents	Adults	Geriatrics	Validation method	Rating (0,1,2)	
								5. Identifies safety concerns.
								a. Identifies age-appropriate safety measures when providing patient care and reports potential safety concerns.
								b. Identifies age-appropriate signs of abuse/neglect and reports to appropriate personnel or community agencies.

Performance narrative

Figure 7.4 — Registered radiologic technologist job description (cont.)

Neonates	Infants	Children	Adolescents	Adults	Geriatrics	Validation method	Rating (0,1,2)

6. Evaluates the patient's responses to care.
   a. Assesses patient for signs of pain and reports appropriately.
   b. Analyzes data to identify ongoing patient care needs.
   c. Modifies plan of care to meet patient's identified needs.

Performance narrative

7. Documents and communicates care.
   a. Documents care provided and patient's response according to policies and procedures.
   b. Documents history on requisition of chief complaint.
   c. Documents LMP on all females ages 12–55 (knees to diaphragms).
   d. Documents fluoroscopy time when appropriate on requisition.

Performance narrative

8. Assumes all other duties and responsibilities as necessary.
   a. Accepts leader/charge QC responsibilities appropriate to level of development.
   b. Demonstrates dependability/flexibility in meeting scheduling needs of the unit.
   c. Accepts assignment as preceptor of new staff.

Performance narrative

Figure 7.4 — Registered radiologic technologist job description (cont.)

Unit-specific core competencies: diagnostic radiology

Neonates	Infants	Children	Adolescents	Adults	Geriatrics	Validation method	Rating (0,1,2)	
								1. Demonstrates care of the patient with supportive devices.
								a. Cervical Collar.
								b. Backboard.
								c. Traction Devices.

Performance narrative

Neonates	Infants	Children	Adolescents	Adults	Geriatrics	Validation method	Rating (0,1,2)	
								2. Identifies and implements care specific to radiation protection.
								a. Demonstrates lead shielding.
								b. Demonstrates proper collimation.

Performance narrative

Neonates	Infants	Children	Adolescents	Adults	Geriatrics	Validation method	Rating (0,1,2)	
								3. Portable machines.
								a. Able to operate equipment and obtain portable radiographs.
								b. Secure key in locked box in accordance with ODH and Joint Commission..

Performance narrative

Neonates	Infants	Children	Adolescents	Adults	Geriatrics	Validation method	Rating (0,1,2)	
								4. Fluoroscopy equipment
								a. Manages equipment.
								b. Assists physician with procedures.
								c. Documents fluoroscopy time.
								d. Contacts physician as needed.

Performance narrative

Figure 7.4: Registered radiologic technologist job description (cont.)

Employee comments:

[blank text box]

Manager comments:

[blank text box]

I have read this review. Signature does not indicate agreement.

Employee signature:_____ Date:_____

Reviewer's signature:_____ Date:_____

Figure 7.5 — Security officer job description

Date:	Employee number:	Last revision date: 9/2004
Employee name:		Job title: Security Officer
Department:		Reports to: Unit Director
Signatures:		Select one of the following:
		___ Post-orientation competency assessment
Director: _____ Date: _____		___ Other
VP/AVP: _____ Date: _____		

BASIC PURPOSE OF THE JOB

The primary purpose of security services is to provide a safe and secure environment for all employees, physicians, and visitors at _____ Hospital.

CONTACTS

Age of patient populations served *(Check all that apply)*

		Competency validation methods
Neonates (1–30 days)	Adults (19–70 years)	O = Observation/Demonstration
Infants (30 days to 1 year)	Geriatric (>70 years)	PT = Post test
Children (1–12 years)		D = Drills
Adolescents (13–18 years)	No Patient Contact	PI = Performance Improvement Monitors
		E = Exemplars (Examples of feedback that consistently validates knowledge of competence)

JOB REQUIREMENTS

- High school diploma with security, safety, or police experience
- Associate's degree in criminal justice or related field preferred
- Must possess a valid driver's license and an acceptable driving record
- Strong interpersonal skills with ability to handle a wide variety of circumstances and conditions
- Clearance on background check

WORKING CONDITIONS

- Rotate shifts: works every other weekend and holidays as assigned
- Lunch and break periods are coordinated with other staff to maintain adequate coverage
- Hazard exposure rating: 1
- Subject to frequent interruptions during performance of duties

THE COMPETENCY VALIDATION PROCESS

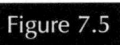

Security officer job description (cont.)

Core competencies/job description

Rating scale and definitions

2 = Consistently exceeds standards	Performance consistently surpasses all established standards. Activities often contribute to improved or innovative work practices. This category is to be used for truly outstanding performance
1 = Consistently meets/sometimes exceeds standards	Performance meets all established standards and sometimes exceeds them. Activities contribute to increased unit results. Employees consistently complete the work that is required and at times go beyond expectations.
0 = Developmental/needs improvement	Performance meets most but not all of established standards. Activities sometimes contribute to unit results. This category is to be used for employees who must demonstrate improvement or more consistent performance and for employees still learning their job. Areas for improvement are included in the narrative.

gray box indicates the activity is not age related, white indicates age-specific

Essential functions

Essential functions are those tasks, duties, and responsibilities that comprise the means of accomplishing the job's purpose and objectives. Essential functions are critical or fundamental to the performance of the job. They are the major functions that the person in the job is held accountable for. Following are the essential functions of the job, along with the corresponding performance standards:

Neonates	Infants	Children	Adolescents	Adults	Geriatrics	Validation method	Rating (0,1,2)	
								1. **Patrol hospital buildings and premises to prevent fire, theft, vandalism, and intruders.**
▓	▓	▓	▓	▓	▓			a. Reports safety/fire hazards to supervisor.
▓	▓	▓	▓	▓	▓			b. Confronts and questions unauthorized persons in a professional manner.
▓	▓	▓	▓	▓	▓			c. Able to control all serious incidents in reference to detainment and eviction of individual(s) not conforming to acceptable standards for visitors, employees, and hospital property
▓	▓	▓	▓	▓	▓			d. Outside security checks: Checks all surface lots, parking deck, dock area exterior doors, and other exterior property on an hourly basis or as designated by the lead shift officer.
▓	▓	▓	▓	▓	▓			e. Inside security checks: Checks all nursing floors, interior doors, and all other miscellaneous floors throughout the hospital on an hourly basis or as designated by the lead shift officer.
▓	▓	▓	▓	▓	▓			f. Maintains traffic flow in an organized manner and enforces parking regulations.
▓	▓	▓	▓	▓	▓			g. Upon request, escorts personnel to parking lots and hospital buildings in a safe and professional manner.
▓	▓	▓	▓	▓	▓			h. Handles all requested monetary transactions in a safe and efficient manner.
▓	▓	▓	▓	▓	▓			I. Handles vehicle accidents and incidents in an appropriate manner.
▓	▓	▓	▓	▓	▓			j. Performs jump starts, vehicle unlocks, and moves vehicles as required.

Performance narrative

Figure 7.5 — Security officer job description (cont.)

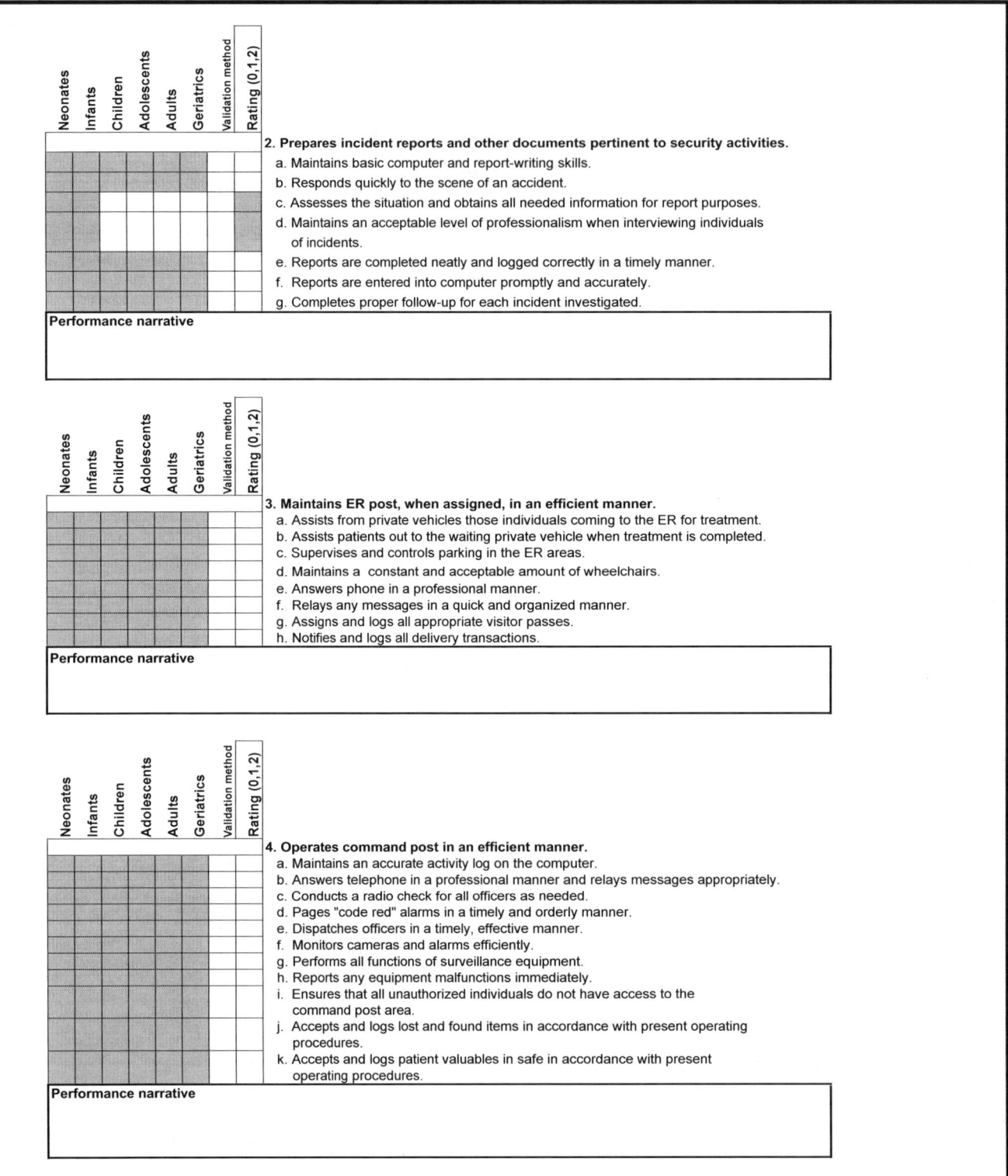

Columns: Neonates | Infants | Children | Adolescents | Adults | Geriatrics | Validation method | Rating (0,1,2)

2. Prepares incident reports and other documents pertinent to security activities.
   a. Maintains basic computer and report-writing skills.
   b. Responds quickly to the scene of an accident.
   c. Assesses the situation and obtains all needed information for report purposes.
   d. Maintains an acceptable level of professionalism when interviewing individuals of incidents.
   e. Reports are completed neatly and logged correctly in a timely manner.
   f. Reports are entered into computer promptly and accurately.
   g. Completes proper follow-up for each incident investigated.

Performance narrative

3. Maintains ER post, when assigned, in an efficient manner.
   a. Assists from private vehicles those individuals coming to the ER for treatment.
   b. Assists patients out to the waiting private vehicle when treatment is completed.
   c. Supervises and controls parking in the ER areas.
   d. Maintains a constant and acceptable amount of wheelchairs.
   e. Answers phone in a professional manner.
   f. Relays any messages in a quick and organized manner.
   g. Assigns and logs all appropriate visitor passes.
   h. Notifies and logs all delivery transactions.

Performance narrative

4. Operates command post in an efficient manner.
   a. Maintains an accurate activity log on the computer.
   b. Answers telephone in a professional manner and relays messages appropriately.
   c. Conducts a radio check for all officers as needed.
   d. Pages "code red" alarms in a timely and orderly manner.
   e. Dispatches officers in a timely, effective manner.
   f. Monitors cameras and alarms efficiently.
   g. Performs all functions of surveillance equipment.
   h. Reports any equipment malfunctions immediately.
   i. Ensures that all unauthorized individuals do not have access to the command post area.
   j. Accepts and logs lost and found items in accordance with present operating procedures.
   k. Accepts and logs patient valuables in safe in accordance with present operating procedures.

Performance narrative

Figure 7.5 — Security officer job description (cont.)

Columns: Neonates | Infants | Children | Adolescents | Adults | Geriatrics | Validation method | Rating (0,1,2)

5. Will respond to, or page assistance calls as needed (code red, trouble alarms, medical assistance, code yellow, code gray, standby).
 a. Pages all assistance calls accurately and in a timely manner.
 b. Reponds to the assistance calls acccurately and in a timely manner.
 c. Evaluates and controls the situation in an orderly, safe, and professional fashion.

Performance narrative

6. Maintains department equipment in good operating condition.
 a. Drives security vehicles/bicycles in a safe, professional manner.
 b. Keeps vehicles/bicycles clean.
 c. Reports any vehicles/bicycle equipment failures for necessary repairs.
 d. Keeps radios and other equipment in operating condition.

Performance narrative

Employee comments:

Manager comments:

I have read this review. Signature does not indicate agreement.

Employee signature:_____ Date:_____

Reviewer's Signature:_____ Date:_____

Chapter seven

Figure 7.6 | **Ongoing competency assessment, Sample 1**

Ongoing competency assessment

Employee name: Angela Caldwell—UD   **Date:**

Department: Memorial 5 South   **Job title:** Registered Nurse

Mandated competencies	Yes	No	Validation method
1.			
2.			
3.			

New/changed competencies

Columns: Complete(Y/N), Neonates, Infants, Children, Adolescents, Adults, Geriatric, Validation method, Date, Initials

1. Implementation of natrecore protocol
2. CDC hand hygiene
3. Biphasic monitoring (synchronized cardioversion and ext. pacing)

Low-volume/high-risk competencies

Columns: Complete(Y/N), Neonates, Infants, Children, Adolescents, Adults, Geriatric, Validation method, Date, Initials

1. Restraints
2. Endotracheal tube and tracheostomy suctioning
3. Transmission-driven isolation set-up and communication

Problem-prone competencies

Columns: Complete(Y/N), Neonates, Infants, Children, Adolescents, Adults, Geriatric, Validation method, Date, Initials

1. Chest tubes—Source: PI variances
2. Pain—Source: Patient satisfaction
3. Customer Service—Source: Pt. satisfaction

This employee continues to demonstrate the core competencies by virtue of no aggregate data source to identify otherwise.   Yes_____ No_____

Sources:
1. Quality reports
2. Patient perception report
3. Other reports

Manager signature _____   Date _____

Competency validator _____   Date _____

Validation Grid: PT = Post-test   PI = Performance improvement monitors
D = Drills   E = Exemplars (Examples of feedback that consistently
O = Observation/return demonstration   validates knowledge of competency)

THE COMPETENCY VALIDATION PROCESS

Figure 7.7 — Ongoing competency assessment, Sample 2

Ongoing Competency Assessment

Employee name: _____ **Date:** _____

Department: Radiology   **Job title:** RADIOLOGIC TECHNOLOGIST
Billie Rotunno—UD

Organization-mandated competencies	Yes	No	Validation method
1. Safety education			
2. CPR			
3. National patient safety goals			
4. TB			

Departmental-mandated competencies
1. Selects appropriate technical factors "ALARA"
2. Performs procedure types in accordance with protocols
3. Correct type and dosage of contrast material

New/changed competencies

Columns: Complete(Y/N) | Neonates | Infants | Children | Adolescents | Adults | Geriatric | Validation method | Date | Initials

1. Implementation of Fuji CR computers
2. CDC hand hygiene

Low volume/high risk competencies

Columns: Complete(Y/N) | Neonates | Infants | Children | Adolescents | Adults | Geriatric | Validation method | Date | Initials

1. Pediatric IVP exams
2. Pediatric GI/BE exams

Problem-prone competencies

Columns: Complete(Y/N) | Neonates | Infants | Children | Adolescents | Adults | Geriatric | Validation method | Date | Initials

1. Repeat rate: PI variance
2. LMP documentation: PI variance

This employee continues to demonstrate the core competencies
by virtue of no aggregate data source to identify otherwise.   Yes_____ No_____

Sources:
1. Quality reports
2. Patient perception report
3. Other reports

Manager signature _____ Date _____

Competency validator _____ Date _____

Validation grid:
- PT = Post-test
- D = Drills
- O = Observation/return demonstration
- PI = Performance improvement monitors
- E = Exemplars (examples of feedback that consistently validates knowldege of competency)

COMPETENCY ASSESSMENT, THIRD EDITION

Figure 7.8: Ongoing competency assessment, Sample 3

Ongoing competency assessment

Employee name: _____ Date: _____

Department: **Security services**   Job title: **Security Officer**

Mandated competencies

	Yes	No	Validation method

Competency	Complete (Y/N)	Neonates	Infants	Children	Adolescents	Adults	Geriatric	Validation method	Date	Initials
Code red (Fire)								D/O		
Lifts/carries								O/PI		
Extinguisher use								O/PI		
Fire hose								O		
Code Adam								D/O		
Self-defense								O		
Restraints								O		
Vehicle extrication								O		

New/changed competencies

Competency	Complete (Y/N)	Neonates	Infants	Children	Adolescents	Adults	Geriatric	Validation method	Date	Initials
Concealed weapons								O		

Low-volume/high-risk competencies

Competency	Complete (Y/N)	Neonates	Infants	Children	Adolescents	Adults	Geriatric	Validation method	Date	Initials
Code orange (spills)								D/O		
Code black (bomb)								D/O		

Problem-prone competencies

Competency	Complete (Y/N)	Neonates	Infants	Children	Adolescents	Adults	Geriatric	Validation method	Date	Initials
Customer service: Source–Emp. exchange Patient satisfaction								Data analysis/E		

Sources:
1. Quality reports
2. Patient perception report
3. Other reports

Manager signature _____   Date _____

Competency validator _____   Date _____

Validation grid: PT = Post-test   PI = Performance improvement monitors
D = Drills   E = Exemplars (examples of feedback that consistently
O = Observation/return demonstration   validates knowledge of competency)

Figure 7.9 — Annual performance evaluation: Organizational competencies

Employee Name: _____
Employee Number: _____
Department: _____
Date: _____
Position: _____

Rating Scale and Definitions

2 = Consistently Exceeds Standards	Performs consistently surpasses all established standards. Activities oftern contribute to improved or innovative work practices. This category is to be used for truly outstanding performance
1 = Consistently Meets/Sometimes Exceeds Standards	Performance meets all established standards and sometimes exceeds them. Activities contribute to increased unit results. Employees consistently complete the work that is required and at times go beyond expectations.
0 = Developmental/Needs Improvement	Performance meets most, but not all, established standards. Activities sometimes contribute to unit results. This category is to be used for employees who must demonstrate improvement or more consistent performance and for employees still learning their job. Areas for improvement are included in the narrative.

Figure 7.9 | **Annual performance evaluation: Organizational competencies (cont.)**

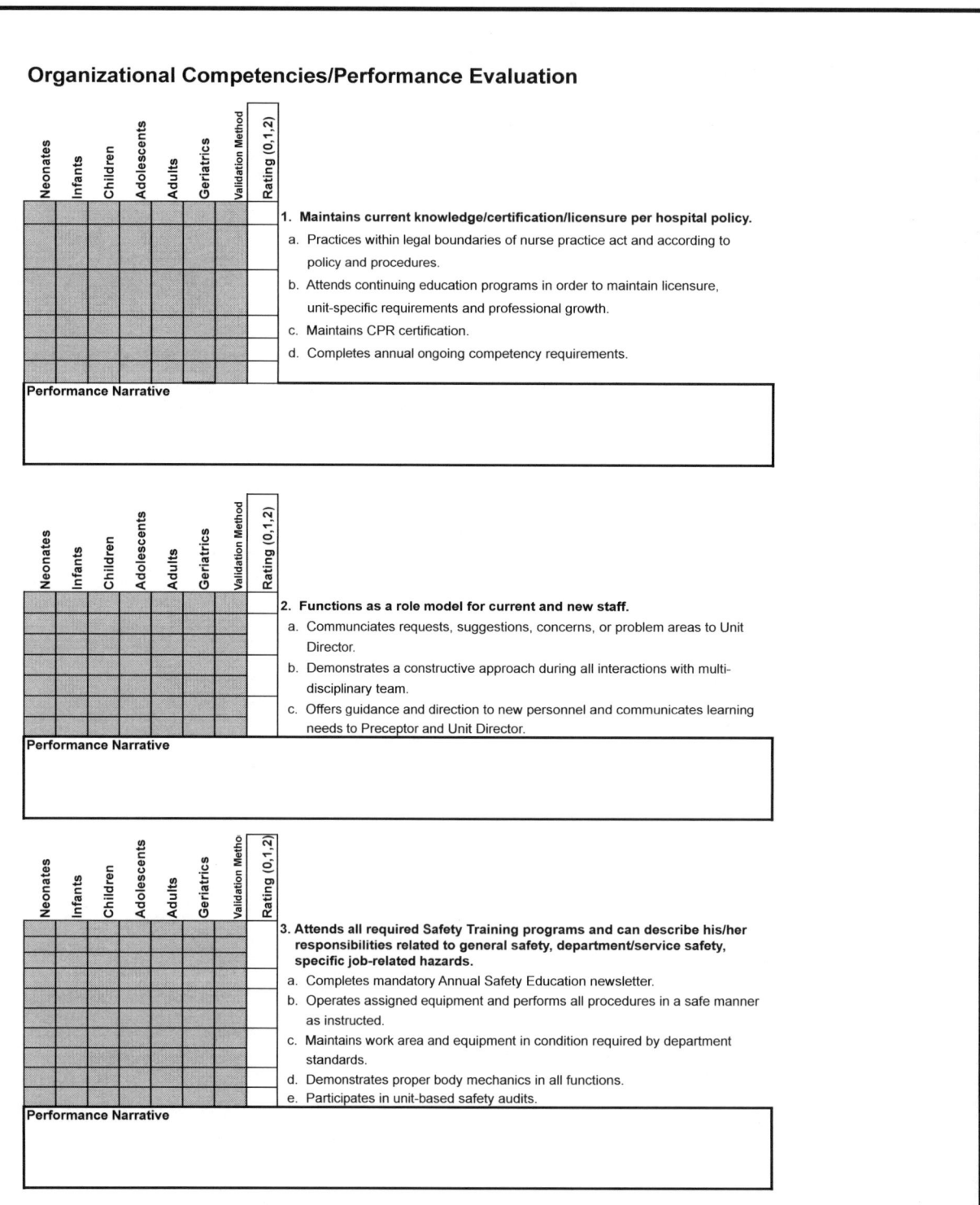

Figure 7.9 — Annual performance evaluation: Organizational competencies (cont.)

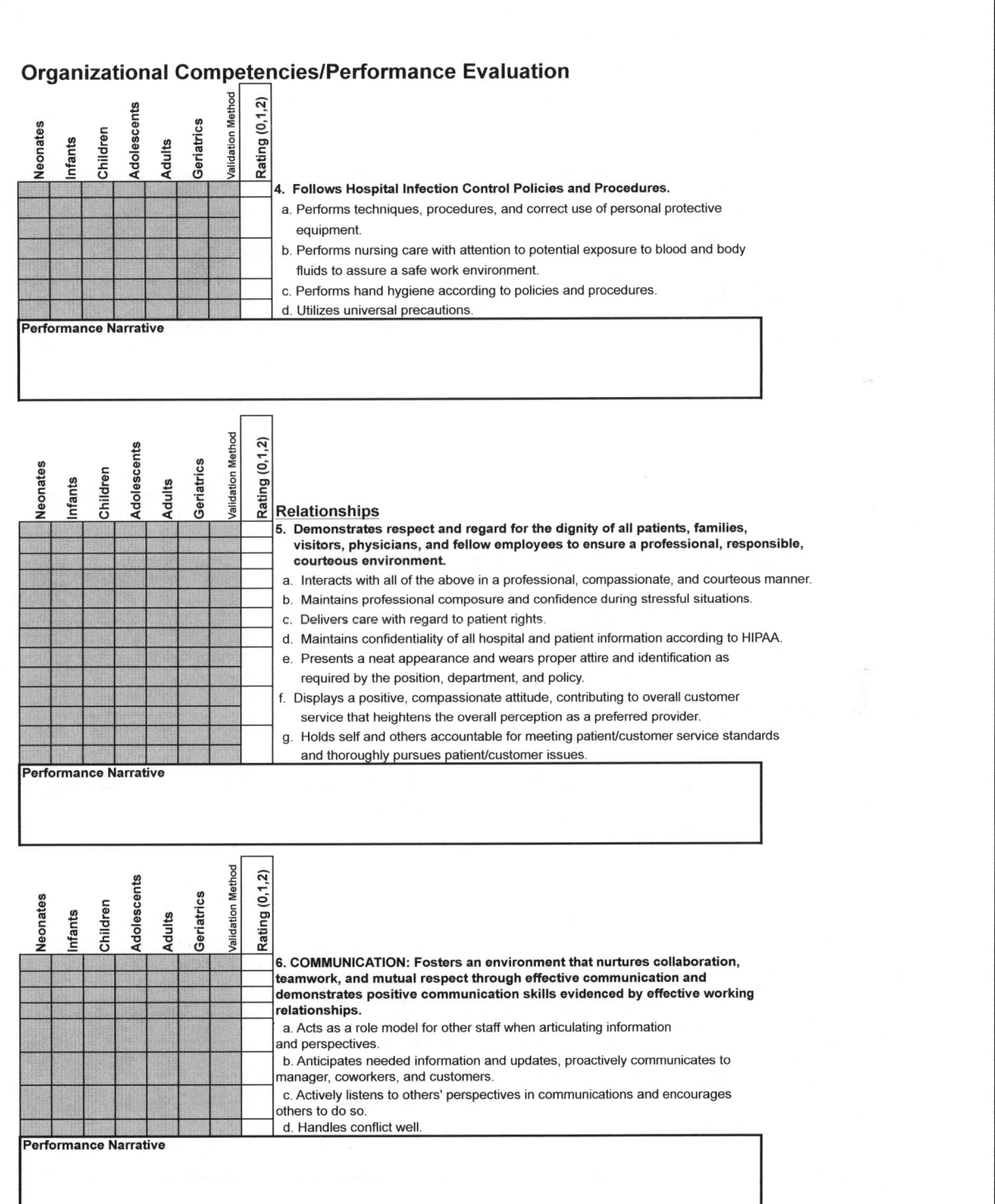

Organizational Competencies/Performance Evaluation

4. Follows Hospital Infection Control Policies and Procedures.
 a. Performs techniques, procedures, and correct use of personal protective equipment.
 b. Performs nursing care with attention to potential exposure to blood and body fluids to assure a safe work environment.
 c. Performs hand hygiene according to policies and procedures.
 d. Utilizes universal precautions.

Performance Narrative

Relationships
5. Demonstrates respect and regard for the dignity of all patients, families, visitors, physicians, and fellow employees to ensure a professional, responsible, courteous environment.
 a. Interacts with all of the above in a professional, compassionate, and courteous manner.
 b. Maintains professional composure and confidence during stressful situations.
 c. Delivers care with regard to patient rights.
 d. Maintains confidentiality of all hospital and patient information according to HIPAA.
 e. Presents a neat appearance and wears proper attire and identification as required by the position, department, and policy.
 f. Displays a positive, compassionate attitude, contributing to overall customer service that heightens the overall perception as a preferred provider.
 g. Holds self and others accountable for meeting patient/customer service standards and thoroughly pursues patient/customer issues.

Performance Narrative

6. COMMUNICATION: Fosters an environment that nurtures collaboration, teamwork, and mutual respect through effective communication and demonstrates positive communication skills evidenced by effective working relationships.
 a. Acts as a role model for other staff when articulating information and perspectives.
 b. Anticipates needed information and updates, proactively communicates to manager, coworkers, and customers.
 c. Actively listens to others' perspectives in communications and encourages others to do so.
 d. Handles conflict well.

Performance Narrative

Figure 7.9 Annual performance evaluation: Organizational competencies (cont.)

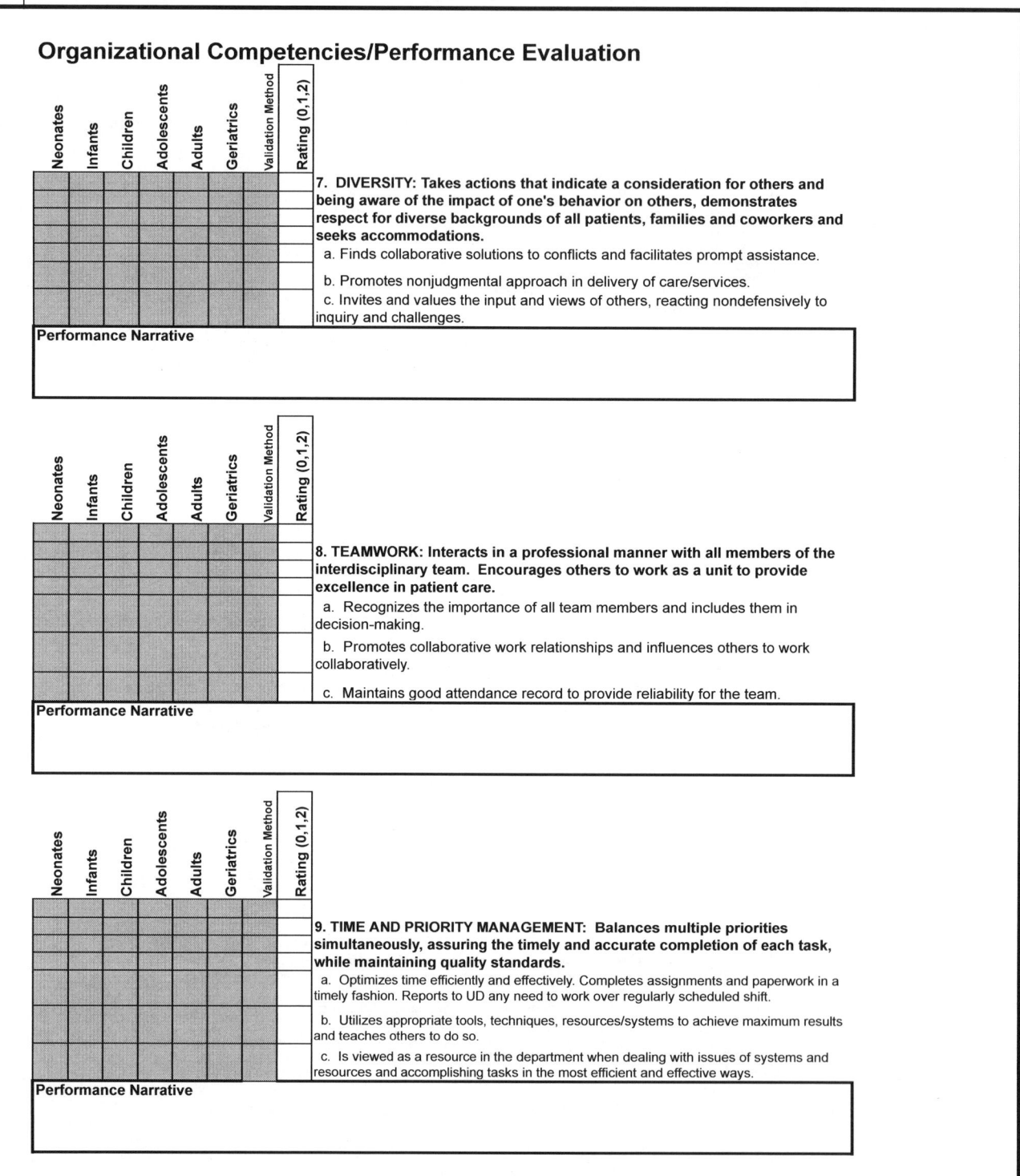

Figure 7.9 — **Annual performance evaluation: Organizational competencies (cont.)**

Organizational Competencies/Performance Evaluation

Progress Toward Previous Year's Goals

Goals for Next Evaluation Period:

Employee Comments:

Manager Comments:

I have read this review. Signature does not indicate agreement.

Employee Signature:_____ **Date:**_____

Reviewer's Signature:_____ **Date:**_____

Chapter eight

Managing the competency program

Managing the competency program

Like any process, the competency validation process must be managed by someone: an individual or a group of individuals. There are activities that must be completed each year and those that must be managed during the year. The process can best be represented as a continuum, with components but no actual beginning or end. An analogy that many in healthcare will recognize is that of the budget process, which is really a continuum itself. Neither the competency process nor the budget process is one that can be addressed if the leaders walk away from it, as if the process were complete and no further attention were needed.

Getting started

Take the following four steps to get the competency validation process started:

1. Assign responsibility for the process to an individual or to a group of people knowledgeable about the competency process and the tools used at the organization.

2. Create a work calendar with timelines.

3. Decide on a competency validation tool/format that can be used for all staff.

4. Populate the tool (involve staff that actually perform the job).

  - Rules for populating the competency validation tool, **always beginning with the template for newly hired staff:**
    - Review job responsibilities/activities/competencies for **all** newly employed staff in a **specific job group/job title** (Part 1/Level I, all job responsibilities/activities/competencies [i.e., all physical therapists, all registrars, all housekeepers, all security officers, all insurance verifiers, all coders, all registered nurses, etc.]).

Chapter eight

Chapter eight

- Add each job responsibility/activity/competency to the validation tool.

- Use verbs (e.g., assesses _____, administers medications, plans care, cleans _____, obtains patient demographic information, etc.). Rule: You cannot validate the verbs "understands" or "knows."

- If reviewing a clinical job, follow the clinical process: Assess, plan, and intervene, and include patient/family education when populating the validation tool.

- Identify all responsibilities/activities/competencies that have an age/population-related aspect to them and highlight them in some way, such as the use of bold font, different-color font, etc.

- Determine whether there are "rules" (i.e., policies, procedures, protocols, etc.) for how the responsibilities/activities/competencies are to be completed, including how they are to be altered, if age/population-related.

- Assign the development of rules to a subgroup, if they are not already available or if they need modification.

• Note that it is unusual to have a job group that goes beyond the level of Part III.

- Look across all the identified job responsibilities/activities/competencies found in the job description and on the competency validation tool for new employees, noting all those performed by more than one discipline/job group.

- Ensure rules and tools are the same for all staff members performing the same responsibilities/activities/competencies.

- Identify additional (i.e., unit/population-specific) responsibilities, if there are any, and add them to the template as Part II/Level II responsibilities/activities/competencies. This can cover all physical therapists in the nursery, all registered nurses in home care, all registrars in the ED, etc.

- Identify additional (i.e., unit/population-specific) responsibilities, if there are any, and add them to the template as Part III/Level III responsibilities/activities/competencies. This can cover all registered nurses in the critical care units, cardiac ICU, all physical therapists, nursery, neonatal transport team, etc.

- Identify the appropriate competency validation method(s) and add them to the tool in the designated column.

- Determine whether validation "tools" already exist; if not, assign their development to a subgroup and include someone in the group who has expertise in the use of the different validation methods.

• Determine those qualified to validate competency, noting that this will likely vary by job title/job group.

• Begin using the process to validate competency for all newly hired staff.

Ongoing competency

Consider the following tips as you review for ongoing competency:

• Review aggregate data sources on an ongoing basis. These data may indicate either continued competency in how staff members are carrying out the primary responsibilities/activities/competencies of the job, or they may indicate a problem with how some or all of the staff members are carrying out aspects of their jobs.

• Review job responsibilities/activities/competencies for **all newly employed** staff in a **specific job group/job title** (Part 1, all ___ job responsibilities/activities/competencies [e.g., all physical therapists, all registrars, all housekeepers, all security officers, all insurance verifiers, all coders, all registered nurses, etc.])

• Ask four questions about the responsibilities/activities/competencies identified for newly hired staff:

- Are any responsibilities/activities/competencies **low volume**?

- Are any responsibilities/activities/competencies scheduled to change in the way they have been done OR are there responsibilities/activities/competencies scheduled to be added to the job responsibilities (**changed or new**)?

- Are any responsibilities/activities/competencies **mandated by an external regulatory agency** (e.g., CDC, TJC, CMS, OSHA, etc.) for annual education and competency validation, no matter how often they are done or how well they are done?

- Are any responsibilities/activities/competencies those that have been identified through review of aggregate data as being **problem prone**?

- If the answer is "yes" about any responsibility/activity/competency on the new employee list, add this responsibility/activity/competency to the list of those requiring education/re-education and competency validation by current staff. Use the wording exactly as it appears on the template for newly hired staff. The same considerations regarding age/population-related aspects of the job, rules and tools, and validation method(s) apply here as well.

- Ask the four questions about all levels/parts, as the answers may differ when asked about the responsibilities/activities/competencies assigned to the different parts/levels.

• Begin using the process to validate ongoing competency for all current staff.

Ongoing competency statement

For many jobs, the answer to the four questions is "no" to each. In this situation, the employee demonstrates ongoing competency every day he or she comes to work and performs, with a degree of regularity, the unchanged aspects of his or her job. No one is lucky enough to frequently perform activities incompetently and not have it be identified through a review of aggregate data reports. In this case, a statement to this effect is all that is needed for the documentation of ongoing competency (see Figure 8.1). For others, it is the ongoing competency statement, plus one or more of the responsibility/activities/competencies added to the list for annual education and competency validation, plus the ongoing competency statement.

Figure 8.1 | **Ongoing competency statement**

_____ continues to demonstrate competency in all high-volume, unchanged, nonmandated aspects of the job by virtue of no data source indicating otherwise.

_____   _____
Leader's signature   Date

Maintenance of the process

Just as a new budget must be developed and monitored at least monthly, so must the competency process. Leaders must review the aggregate data reports available to them, to both identify ongoing competency of staff, and to identify problem-prone aspects of the different jobs performed by staff members reporting to them.

Provide staff members with education on all the topics identified on the ongoing competency templates, using outside resources if needed, and then validate ongoing competency using the same method(s) used for newly hired staff.

Accommodate unplanned additions to the ongoing competency validation plans during the year if they arise. These could include unplanned changes to a current job responsibility/activity, the addition of new responsibilities, or problems in how staff members are performing a primary responsibility/activity of the job.

The same individual or group charged with getting the process started should be the person or group who ensures continued maintenance of the process. Figure 8.2 shows the charter and yearly planning calendar for a group in one hospital charged with this responsibility.

Chapter Eight

Figure 8.2 — **Competency Management Council**

Competency assessment is an ongoing process that exists over the continuum of the employment/work experience:

HIRE   **INITIAL**   **ONGOING**

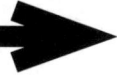

The competency process must address the unique requirements of each phase. This process is dynamic and addresses the needs of each phase separately.

- ***Prior to hire***, base competency is assessed through licensure/registration/certification, previous experience, education/training, and interview questions directed at behavioral and functional requirements of the job.

- ***Initial*** job competencies are assessed during the orientation and observation prior to independent functioning in the job role.

- ***Ongoing*** competency assessment is a dynamic process based on the fluid needs required to carry out the organization's mission and strategic goals. These requirements are based on: 1) mandated regulations, 2) low-volume/high-risk activities, 3) problem-prone activities, or 4) new/changed aspects of a job.

Charter:

- The Competency Management Council will provide a multidisciplinary approach to managing the competency assessment process within the <u>Hospital Name</u> organization.

- The council will be responsible for general oversight of the competency process for both "new hire" and "ongoing" competency documents. This responsibility includes oversight of:
  - The initial development documents for existing jobs and any jobs that are created in the future
  - Updates to completed documents in the competency repository
  - Retirement of documents that are no longer pertinent to the organization
  - The validation of rules and tools for all documents

> **Figure 8.2** — **Competency Management Council (cont.)**
>
> - The council will collaborate with department leaders to identify necessary annual or interim competency adjustments based on data analysis results.
>
> - The council will present to the administrative council the annual report of organizational competency and the organizational plan for annual competency assessment in January of each year.
>
> *Membership:*
> - HR Generalists (2)
> - Manager, Clinical Education
> - Clinical Nurse Specialist
> - Clinical Educator, Radiology
> - Clinical Educator
> - Clinical Instructor
> - Nursing Informatics
> - Educator reps:
>   - Rehab Services
>   - EVS
>   - Safety
>   - Financial Services
>
> *Initial activities of the Competency Management Council*
>
> 1. Appoint council chair by ___/___/___ (date TBD)
>
> 2. Council to meet as a group within one week of appointment of council chair

> **Figure 8.2** — **Competency Management Council (cont.)**

3. Council will analyze newly created competency documents:

    • Does each behavior/job function have a correlating *rule*?

    • For each rule for the associated behavior/job function, is there a *tool* to determine validation?

4. Rules and tools for each job to be listed in the repository

5. Council to coordinate creation of rules and tools using experts

6. Council to determine "go live" date and transition plans for the competency management processes

Timeline of annual activities of the Competency Management Council

Month	Activities
January	• Council presents to administrative council the annual report of organizational competency and the organizational plan for annual competency assessment • Education calendar for upcoming year published/distributed • Schedule appointments with each department for upcoming year to review "new" and "ongoing" competency documents
February	• Review "new" and "ongoing" competency documents per schedule set in January
March	• Quarterly meetings with department leaders for data reports influencing competency planning
April	• Review "new" and "ongoing" competency documents per schedule set in January
May	• No activity scheduled

Figure 8.2 — Competency Management Council (cont.)

June	• Quarterly meetings with department leaders for data reports influencing competency planning
July	• Review "new" and "ongoing" competency documents per schedule set in January
August	• Department leaders to gather information for ongoing competency needs
September	• Annual meetings with each department leader/representative to discuss ongoing competency needs to determine education plan for upcoming year
October	• Review "new" and "ongoing" competency documents per schedule set in January
November	• Quarterly meetings with department leaders for data reports influencing competency planning; finalization of upcoming educational plan for each department
December	• Finalization of upcoming educational plan for each department

A review of the calendar shows that each year the cycle begins anew. Without administrative support for maintenance of the competency process, there will be a great flurry of activity in the beginning, and then a return to the old way of doing things, in an effort to fill the void created by the transition to the newly designed process.